Methodology
of
Traditional Chinese Medicine

Huang Jianping

New World Press, Beijing, China

First Edition 1995

Copyright by **New World Press,** Beijing, China. All rights reserved. No part of this book may be reproduced in any form or by any means without permission in writing from the publisher.

ISBN 7-80005-266-4

Published by
NEW WORLD PRESS
24 Baiwanzhuang Road, Beijing 100037, China

Distributed by
CHINA INTERNATIONAL BOOK TRADING CORPORATION
35 Chegongzhuang Xilu, Beijing 100044, China
P.O. Box 399, Beijing, China

Printed in the People's Republic of China

CONTENTS

Chapter I
MEDICAL SCIENCE AND TECHNOLOGY ... 5
Difference in Methodology Between Chinese and Western Medicine ... 8
Systematics, Cybernetics and Informatics and Methodology of Chinese Medicine ... 15

Chapter II
THE YIN-YANG THEORY ... 22
Genesis ... 22
Integration of Yin and Yang ... 24
The *Wuxing* Theory and Order in the Human Body ... 42
Interrelation Between Nature and Mankind in the Yin-Yang Theory ... 52
Study of the Yin-Yang Theory in Modern Medicine ... 61
The Yin-Yang Theory in Chinese Medicine ... 68

Chapter III
THE *ZANGXIANG* THEORY ... 71
Genesis ... 71
Tentative Comment on "Reverberating View of Inside Scene" ... 79
The *Zangxiang* Theory from the Viewpoint of Yin and Yang ... 84

Chapter IV
THE *BIANZHENGLUNZHI* THEORY ... 102
Genesis ... 102
Bianzheng and Treatment ... 106
Scrutinizing Syndromes to Search for the Cause of Disease ... 123
Traditional Methods of Diagnosing Symptoms ... 129
Methodology in the Principles of Treatment ... 136

Chapter V
THE SCIENTIFIC SIGNIFICANCE OF TRADITIONAL METHODOLOGY ... 152

Chapter VI
SIGNIFICANCE OF THEORY AND METHOD IN CHINESE MEDICINE ... 159
Presentation of the Problem ... 159

Characteristics of Chinese Medicine and Its Trend	161
The Training of Chinese Medical Personnel	172
The Promotion of Research and Practice	180
NOTES	186
INDEX	188

Chapter I

MEDICAL SCIENCE AND TECHNOLOGY

Whenever we conduct scientific research or engage in any medical practice— consciously or unconsciously, we adopt a certain method. That is, we adopt a means or procedure in order to attain our goals. Methodology is a theory or rationale concerning this procedure of reaching goals. It takes the method, or means, as its object and studies the basic rules and laws governing various methods. The term "methodology" might be defined as a rationale of laws concerning a method.

Some believe that a method is something one can choose at his own discretion and that there is no need to follow, learn or study a specific one. Others believe that the most expedient method for reaching a goal is also the best. For instance, physicist Ernst Mach (1838-1916) advocated the "principle of economic thinking," maintaining that man should think "most economically," regardless of what the consequences might be. According to Mach, the best methods are those by which the goal is reached most expediently and pragmatically. This shows that a method is only something created at will by human intelligence; it needs to follow no other guidelines than those set by the individual. But is this point of view correct?

Daily life and work may answer the question. In the realm of human society, the exploitation of one country could certainly be regarded as a most expedient and practical way for another to get rich. But at what cost for those exploited? For them, it would be catastrophic. In nature, one cannot deny that "draining the pond to get all the fish" is a most expedient and practical way to catch them, but it would spoil future resources. Felling trees in large quantities is also an expedient way of obtaining lumber; again, the ecological repercussions would be disastrous, resulting in barren hills, erosion, and the upsetting of nature's equilibrium. Evidently, clinging to one's own way and disregarding objective laws, a person will eventually fail in what he attempts to do.

That is also true with medical practice. Some doctors, who are not versed in medicine, usually give treatment to their patients before making a good analysis of their symptoms, constitution and case histories. No wonder that they make errors in treatment, thus lessening the chances of a patient's recovery or further endangering his health.

Zhang Zhongjing (150-219), a doctor of the late Han Dynasty (206 B.C.-220 A.D.) known as the "Saint of Medicine," made the following comment:

> It seems to me that physicians nowadays fail to look into medical science and improve their medical skills. Instead, following the same way as their ancestors in practice and adhering to the old therapies, these physicians examine patients and listen to their complaints, and all of them give basis for their treatment. After quick consultation, a plan for treatment is worked out. When they feel the radial artery for the pulse, their fingers are usually improperly placed on both the *cun* (inch) and *chi*[1] (cubit loci) pulses; when they feel wrist pulses, they neglect those on the feet, and leave the condition of the common carotid pulsations[2], the dorsal pedal pulsations[3], and the three regions of the body[4] unconsidered, the number of pulsations and the counts of respiration unascertained, the nine nodes of the pulse[5] and the nose, the forehead and the different parts of the face unexamined. That is the so-called "looking at a leopard through a bamboo tube." A practice like this would certainly make it difficult to discriminate be-

tween life and death.

Evidently, medical experts, whether today or in earlier times, share this view.

Some scientists follow the scientific method of seriously examining and studying a certain feature of an organism or a particular point in its development, and thereby succeed in recognizing all of its details. Often, however, they focus on one aspect to the neglect of the whole process or the entire organism. They end up being conversant with one detail but not with the whole. Consequently, they lack a sufficient grasp or understanding of the organism. In their understanding of only a part, their inferences, assumptions and conclusions about the whole remain flawed.

We maintain that the only correct method of objective study is one which reflects the law of objective things and adopts the proper means to solve problems according to the law. Chinese medicine has always emphasized that the theory, the principle of treatment[6] and the prescription of drugs constitute an inseparable whole. The theory is based on the law of medical science, which in turn produces the principle of treatment or methodology. It is according to the theory and principle of treatment that we work out correct prescriptions and give effective treatment to patients.

There are various things in the world and many methods of identifying them and solving the problems arisen therefrom. The things are different from one another, but their origin is almost the same, such as the diversity and the unity of matter as well as the law of material attraction and repulsion. This shows that all the things in the world have common basic laws and, too, methods applicable to all of them.

Philosophy is a system of knowledge which generalizes the most common laws. The method of thought which reflects these laws is the method that should be learned and mastered in any kind of work. It is called materialistic dialectics. This method, of course, cannot replace actual experience employed in the various departments of science. It is, however, the broad principle guiding the actual methods of various branches of science.

Once this general principle is mastered, we will not miss the forest for the trees and be misled in our basic orientation by committing errors of principles. If the methodology of the various departments of science is to be a proper guide, it must be built on materialistic dialectics, which offers a universal system of guidance. For a medical scientist, familiarity with, and practice of this methodology is crucial.

Difference in Methodology Between Chinese and Western Medicine

Historical differences lead to differences in the recognition of the laws of objective matter. Consequently, different kinds of methods have arisen in different historical periods, occupying dominant positions in their respective times. This is deeply reflected in the methodology of medical science.

Chinese medicine developed under conditions similar to those discussed by Fredrich Engels (1820-1895). He wrote: "Among the Greeks— just because they were not yet advanced enough to dissect, analyze nature— nature is still viewed as a whole, in general. The universal connections of natural phenomena is not proved in regard to particulars; to the Greeks, it is the result of direct contemplation. Herein lies the inadequacy of Greek philosophy, on account of which it had to yield later to other modes of outlook on the world. But herein also lies its superiority over subsequent metaphysical opponents. If in regard to the Greeks, metaphysics was right in particulars, in regard to metaphysics the Greeks were right in general."

When Chinese medicine appeared, social production and division of labor were still underdeveloped. In addition, culture and science had not reached a stage where people needed to dissect and analyze nature. The Chinese were more likely to intuit natural relations and connections. Under such conditions, when dealing with physiology and pathology, Chinese medicine was more likely to view nature and man's place in it holistically. They perceived their interrelations, the unity of opposites in contradiction, and the process of development and change. One can readily see that this holistic concept of the unity of yin and yang, of development and change and of interrelations and reciprocal conditioning has permeated the yin-yang theory; its influence can also be seen in the *zangxiang*[7] (visceral manifestations) and *bianzhenglunzhi* (rendering treatment in accordance with symptoms and signs) theories. Holism in fact amounts to a naive materialist dialectical method.

As Engels pointed out, the overall connections in Chinese medicine have not yet been investigated or explained by modern science. This presents us with a clear and definite task in developing Chinese medicine. While inheriting and further developing its holism and dialectic thought, we should try to study its various aspects in detail and carry on more research by means of modern science and technology.

After the rise and development of an early form of capitalism in Europe, the natural sciences were gradually freed from medieval religious thought. Scientists observed and recorded things as they were, but failed to study the past and development of things and the connections between one thing and another. In order to learn more about a particular thing, they usually worked on one thing and compared its difference with other things, without taking their relations into account.

These methods— isolating one thing from others and paying little attention to the development of one thing— were characteristic of science in its early stages. As Engels pointed out:

> The analysis of nature in its individual parts, the division of the different natural processes and objects into definite classes, the study of the internal anatomy

of organic bodies in their manifold forms— these were the fundamental strides in our knowledge of nature that have been made during the last four hundred years. But this has bequeathed to us the habit of observing natural phenomena and processes in isolation, detached from their general contest; of observing them not in motion but in a state of rest, not as essentially variable elements but as constant one; not in their life but in their death. And when this way of looking at things was transferred by Francis Bacon (1561-1626) and John Locke (1632-1704) from natural science to philosophy, it begot the narrow, metaphysical mode of thought peculiar to the last centuries.

As a branch of natural science, Western medicine has also adopted a metaphysical way of thinking. It played an important role in the early development of medicine in learning about the structure and function of the human body part by part and studying the symptoms and causes of a disease and its method of treatment. This may be evidenced by Andreas Vesalius (1514-1564) who made a study of human anatomy when he divided the human body into several parts and observed them one by one. His work, *The Seven Books on the Structure of the Human Body*, exploded the religious belief in God's creation of life, thus declaring the appearance of modern medicine. Thereafter, following the development of natural science and technology[8], medical science has advanced by the observation and study of the human organism according to its various anatomical patterns.

When it became necessary to study things more closely because of their obvious connections and similarities, metaphysics ran into an opposite extreme and began to obstruct further development in medical science. For instance, Rudolf Virchow (1821-1902), a German pathologist who founded cytopathology, made a great contribution to the description and study of the pathological forms of cells and tissues. Failure came, however, at the point where he attempted to raise conclusive scientific facts to the level of theory.

In his opinion, the extremely complex and varied human body is a union of cells, and a cell as an individual entity has characteristic features that all kinds of life should have and hopes for liberty and autonomy without obeying the common law of the whole. He said that people can acquire an accurate explanation only by discarding mythical unity and looking at each cell as a singular structure and as the cause of life. As for illness, he said, "The essence of an illness is a change in one cell or in a group of cells, and there is no illness other than local illness." He placed stress on local pathological changes but left the reaction of the whole organism to an illness out of account; he paid attention to the *results* of pathological phenomena but ignored their process of *development*.

Research has demonstrated that the local orientation Virchow argued for is incorrect; it does not accurately reflect the connections between local pathological changes and the effect of an illness on the entire body. For example, it was only after the development of the theory of neurohumors that many cases of menopathy, such as functional menorhagia and amenorrhoea, were found to be caused by abnormal periodic changes of the endometrium arising from the disturbance of the functional relations between the cerebral cortex, the hypothalamus, the anterior pituitary and the ovary. If this disease had been diagnosed by studying only the endometrium, it could not have been effectively treated. Only by studying the body holistically and discarding the separatism advocated by metaphysical thought can we recognize the pathological process of complicated interrelations within the body.

Since the latter half of the 19th century, science has moved from the stage of collecting to that of systematizing materials. From the study of the parts, people began to recognize their relationship with the whole organism. Modern medicine could no longer be satisfied with the study of individual organisms, systems or affections. It had to move beyond this to consider the developmental processes involved in organic changes, the relationship between the inside and the outside of the body and the relationship between ecological colonies and individuals within those colonies.

Modern science has begun taking these relationships into account. The development of modern neurophysiology and endocrinology, for instance, has clarified the regulatory function of accommodation and compensation of nerve and body fluids in relation to the whole organism. The development of immunology has elucidated the relationship between causative agents and the body's immune mechanisms. Within the last 30 years, moreover, the study of molecular biology and molecular medicine has cast light on the contradictory movements of an organism. Even these few examples demonstrate the close relationship between the whole and its parts and the attention currently given to this issue.

The development of science demands a truly scientific method. As it has moved from studying isolated parts to looking at the organism holistically, science has turned from metaphysical to dialectic thinking. Engels pointed out that the return from metaphysical thinking, the natural sciences discovering their own strength, would be a long and slow process; he felt that many obstacles would have to be overcome.

Old traditions usually restrict the development of new things. For instance, in his biological research, British scientist Chedd had already recognized the complicated relationship between ribonucleic acid (RNA) and protein. In an article published in the journal *New Science* in 1973, however, he declared notwithstanding that despite its unrivaled complexity, the biological world was no more than the result of the merciless pursuit of self-reproduction of genic molecule. This is obviously incomprehensible. Biological bodies do not just "mercilessly" pursue self-duplication of deoxyribonucleic acid (DNA); instead, DNA will at the same time be transcribed onto ribonucleic acid (RNA) and again undergo the action of the RNA template to translate and manifold proteins. The sequence of RNA-DNA-protein is the process of inheritance and duplication of life. In addition, under the influence of internal and external environments, various elements within an organism can also cause a reaction that can influence RNA under certain conditions. The altered RNA can again counter-transcribe and react on DNA, causing it also to vary; this accounts for variations in living beings. Chedd simplified the rich and varied process of life and took it merely as a process of genetic reproduction. He obviously had not extricated himself from the onesidedness of traditional metaphysics.

In another instance, the recent development of neurophysiology, neuropathology and endocrinology has shown the extremely delicate and important role in anatomy played by the nerve-body fluid neurohumors. The feedback regulation has revealed holistic connections. In modern clinical practice, it is clear that attention needs to be focused on the effect of the neurohumors on other bodily systems. The converse, however, it is that of studying the reactions of other systems and organs on the nerve system, has not been done outside of Chinese medicine. The Chinese practice of considering these things while treating the liver, the spleen, and the kidney[9] has yet to be more fully developed. In the worst case, some people even assume a doubtful or negative attitude toward "illness caused by melancholy," "illness giving rise to melancholy," as well as toward the corresponding regimes of treatment, even though these methods have been effectively practiced in Chinese medicine. Isn't it the force of habit of traditional thinking that has created "unnecessary obstacles" in the development of medicine?

Since it found its way into China more than a century ago, Western medicine has played a significant role in spreading more medical practices and treating diseases. Yet it has been traditional Chinese medicine and medicinal herbs that have protected the health of the masses. By combining Chinese with Western medicine, a new and unified medical science and pharmacology will be created.

Traditional Chinese medicine embodies rich dialectical thought, such as that of the holistic connections and the unity of yin and yang. It deals with many facets of human anatomy and physiology: zang-fu organs[10], jingluo (main and collateral channels), qi (vital energy) and blood, jing (essence of life) and body fluid, the inside and outside of the body, as well as the connections between the whole and the parts. It also examines the effect of the social and natural environment— the universe, the sun and moon, the weather, the seasons and geography on the interrelations and conditioning of yin and yang. The result has been the formation of a system of thought about the interrelations behind spirit and organism, zang and fu, and the inside and outside of the body.

With the development of modern science, medicine has branched out into space medicine, meteorological medicine, environmental medicine and psychosomatic medicine and others. In fact, the ideas of these new sciences can be found in such theories as yin and yang, zangxiang, bianzhenglunzhi, and wuyun and liuqi[11] (five elements' evolutions and six kinds of natural factors), and ziwuliuzhu[12] (midnight-noon ebb-flow). In recent works, scholars have maintained that traditional Chinese medicine contains methodological thought rich in such modern sciences as systematics, cybernetics and informatics. There are many similarities between modern scientific methods and theories on traditional Chinese medicine, though we cannot say that these modern methods have been used in Chinese medicine.

If we look at the issue in its general aspects, however, the aims of traditional Chinese medicine are as follows: to put the human body into a large system for observation and explore the interrelationship among formations, factors and variables, both within and outside the body; to recognize and deal with their interrelations with reference to data that is correspondingly interrelated; to use the principle of stabilization to "harmonize yin and yang to reach a state of equilibrium;" and to readjust their relationship so that they remain in a healthy state.

These aims are the same as those to be reached by modern methodology.

Systematics, Cybernetics and Informatics and Methodology of Chinese Medicine

Probing into such scientific methods as systematics, cybernetics and informatics, and comparing them with the theories on traditional Chinese medicine will make them easily understood.

With the continuing development of science, objects of research are becoming increasingly complicated. In the past, when a researcher tried to learn about a certain thing, he would not have to study various dynamic relations behind it, and its existence could be explained by dealing with the relations between cause and effect, and everything would become clear when he divided it into small parts or elements by dissection and analysis. Things, however, are quite different. When he deals with complicated systems, he has to make thousands of filaments and strands. In so doing, he will find that the relations of cause and effect are no longer direct and linear, but instead are tortuous and complicated in which multiple factors and variables interact upon one another. This shows that the methods prevailing in scientific research a long time ago is out of date, and new methods such as systematics, cybernetics and informatics have appeared over the past 50 years. This trend has played a great role in the development of science.

Half a century ago, the Austrian-Canadian biologist Ludwig von Bertalanffy (1901-   ) said that as more time was spent on individual organs, tissues and molecules, research into the whole became quite obscure, and knowledge about life remained hazy and uncertain. It was for this reason that he proposed that scientific research begin with the whole and devote more time to the biological entity and its surroundings in its entirety. He therefore set up a new branch of science called systematics.

What is a system? In their article *Technology of Organization Management— Systems Engineering* published in the Shanghai-based *Wen Hui Bao* ("Standard") on September 27, 1978, three Chinese scientists Qian Xuesen, Xu Guozhi and Wang Shouyuan asserted: "An extremely complex object of research is usually called a 'system,' which is an organic making a specific function come true through those interacting but interdependent parts. The so-called system itself is a component part of a large-scale system." This shows that a system is an organic entity made up of various individual formations and factors which interact and are related, and is characterized not only by totality and relatedness but by order and dynamism. A systematic method, as Professor Qian Xuesen said, is a one of dealing with a thing in a systematic way. In other words, the interrelation, interaction and restraint between the whole and parts on the one hand, and the entity and its environment on the other are most important.

Created by the U.S. mathematician Norbert Wiener (1894-1964) in 1948, cybernetics has as its subject the generality of structure and the common regularities of control in all systems, whether automatic machines or biological organisms. To control is to carry on readjustment within an organic system according to all changes, internal and external, in order to overcome the indefiniteness of the system, thus preserving its specific features. For instance, if a man wants to live in a constantly changing environment, he must readjust himself to his own organism as well as the environmental changes. The central human control mechanism will have the information obtained analyzed, compared and synthesized so as to make the body take measures in conformity with changes in the environment. During the control process, matter and energy as well as the interrelations of information constitute the entity and a dynamic process takes place. In the process of movement, however, a system is subject to interference at any time by various factors. This interference signals a discrepancy between the controlled quantity and the given or extrinsic one. Control is effected by way of information feedback to change the response to the discrepant signal, bringing about corresponding changes to the controlled quantity as the situation demands in order to eliminate or reduce the discrepancy. The readjustment is realized through the transmission, disposition and feedback of information. Therefore, information is a basic and controlling feature of the control system.

Although information uses matter and energy as a carrier, information itself is neither of these. It generally signifies intelligence, instruction, data, cipher code, signal and related knowledge. Information can be transmitted and sensed directly or indirectly, and is a specific indication of relations between objects. In using information, the concrete pattern assumed by the mater or energy can be ignored; only the informational changes need be noted. Thus, information provides us with a common instrument to study things of different qualities. The method of control consequently crosses the boundary between biological and non-biological entities. It also crosses the line between communication and control, so as to link the different fields of science and make its different systems an integral whole.

The method commonly adopted by systematics, cybernetics and informatics is different from the analytical method mainly used in science before. This new method is characterized by overall synthesis, and attention should be paid to the common regularities in the pattern of motion of matter. With this method, a thing can be recognized and changed in terms of its overall relation to the system. This system may be learned about in an overall entity through synthetic observation from the view of information. No need to perform mechanical recombination after you dissect, analyze and dissolve the internal components of the system one by one as before. All the causes of the system and composite results produced by their interaction can now be studied, not just individual causes and results. The use of input and output replaces the opening of the "black box" as a way to learn about the system; dissection, analysis and reduction are no longer needed. Engels states in his *Dialektik und Natur* ("Dialectics of Nature") states:

> The information method assumes the view point of information and uses information and uses systemic process as process of transmission and switching of information, in which observation of the regularities of movement of a complex system is accomplished through analysis and treatment of the technological process of information. It is different from the traditional empirical method in that it does not sever the relationship of the system. It is also different from mechanical synthesis in that it starts out directly from the overall entity. It is a research method using the viewpoint of relationship and transformation to synthesize the process of the system.

Cybernetics, beginning with the similarities existing universally in nature, discovers the common features among tremendously varied things, and groups them according to what can be analogized and simulated. This lays the foundation for simulating functions. For example, an eagle is a biological thing and an airplane a nonbiological one, but both of them can fly. The reason is that airplane designers have learnt much about flight by studying the eagle. This analogous simulation of function has promoted the rapid development of bionics.

In the black box theory, the internal structure and performance of certain controlled things are thought of as a black box. One method of studying the black box is to dissolve its parts and elements through dissection, analysis and reduction. Opening the black box to learn about its contents is called the "white box" method. However, during the process of opening, the structure and function of the black box itself will often be interfered with and the black box we try to observe is no longer what it used to be, and its original function is hard to understand. Besides, as materialists believe, the formations and elements of things are indefinite. The components inside the black box which we have opened are yet another black box awaiting opening. For instance, thanks to advanced science and technology, molecules and atoms can be opened, but electrons, protons, neutrons and other basic particles, which are also black boxes, still remain to be opened. We are working hard to learn about various things, but what we are confronted with will always be black boxes. For this reason, cybernetics maintains that a method should be discovered of knowing the contents of the black box *without* opening it. By means of this method, we study the relationship between the information put into it and feedback issuing from it, and with feedback and theories on related sciences we can discover the box's contents without opening it. Take for example ultrasonic diagnosis now being used in medicine. With the help of ultrasonic information put into the human body, doctors may get feedback through the different histoid structures or media, which then turns into information image. In so doing, we can make use of the knowledge we have already acquired to find out what *zang* is like without opening the human body's black box.

We see from this that the method and train of thought adopted by systematics, cybernetics and informatics coincide with those of Chinese medicine in many ways. For instance, according to Chinese medicine the human body is a small system in the large-scale system of the universe. This gives rise to the theory of nature-man interrelations. The human body is such a system of different formations and elements in *zang-fu* organs and the *jingluo* system that their balanced and orderly interrelations form an overall entity when the body is in motion. Thus, another theory about *zangxiang* takes shape, dealing with the interrelations between the symptoms of *zang* organs on the one hand, and physical body and mental activity on the other. When yin and yang are in unity along with the body's inter-promotion and restraint and the controlling relationship of feedback regulation— generation, inhibition, restraint and dissolution— among the *zang-fu* organs, the *jingluo* system, *qi* and blood, the human body will then be able to maintain health and stability. Once the orderly relationship between yin and yang is disturbed, a struggle between *qi* and pathogenic factors will ensue. If *qi* is sufficient to regulate itself, health can be preserved; but diseases will set in if there are too many pathogenic factors but too little *qi* to regulate them. At this time, such treating methods as medication, acupuncture, *qigong* (breathing exercise), or massage should be adopted. Deficiency should be treated with tonification to replenish *qi* with excess syndrome being expelled by the purging of pathogenic factors, cold by the warming of the body, and heat by the cooling of the body. Stability is regained and health restored by regulation and control of the opposite side of the confrontation, so as to correct the deviation of yin and yang, and adjust excess or deficiency in generation, inhibition, restraint and dissolution.

In Chinese medicine, the "manifestation" in the *zangxiang* theory is a kind of information about the inner structure and function of the *zang-fu* organs, the *jingluo* system that is expressed externally. *Qi* is a kind of fine and minute matter, and at the same time the carrier of information. With the four methods of diagnosis, a doctor can find out what is wrong with his patient without opening the black box. Then he can give treatment according to the different symptoms and signs, and by summarizing, analyzing and deliberating on the theories used in Chinese medicine. The *zangxiang* and *bianzhenglunzhi* theories, along with pharmacology developed under the guidance of the yin-yang theory, are similar to the theory of the black box. Some scientists also say that treating diseases by means of medication, acupuncture, massage and *qigong* in Chinese medicine is believed to be a "information therapy," namely as direct or indirect input into the body. *Qi* is used as the carrier to act on or readjust yin, yang and the orderly information which has been disturbed. In this respect, there is much that warrants exploration and investigation.

As stated above, systematics, cybernetics and

informatics pay great attention to studying the system holistically. Isomorphism maintains that even matter of different qualities may be simulated or analogized if their states, patterns and functions are similar. Chinese medicine also starts out with the holistic system to adopt methods of simulation and comparison. In this respect, it strikingly resembles systematics, cybernetics and informatics. These methods further develop principles of the dialectics of interrelations, movements and developments. A vast reservoir of dialectic thought is in the theory and methods of Chinese medicine. Consequently, when it is confronted with a very complicated system like that of the human body and the treatment of its disease, it spontaneously develops a great deal of thought similar to that of systematics, cybernetics and informatics. They manifest themselves in naive and plain forms and have much effect on Chinese medical theory and practice. This shows that the Chinese are capable of highly scientific thinking. Thus, if we exert ourselves on this basis and catch up with the times, we will certainly be able to scale the heights of science in the world and make due contributions to mankind.

Over the past 30 years, I have taught philosophy and studied medicine in medical schools, and I have also participated in many clinical practices, including medical treatment. In the course of my scholastic life and medical practice, I have been deeply impressed by the significance of philosophy in medicine, so in this book I will deal with Chinese traditional medicine in three ways: 1) the theory about yin and yang; 2) the theory about the manifestations of *zang*; and 3) *bianzhenglunzhi*. Besides, I will also give my points of view on the trend of Chinese medicine.

Chapter II

THE YIN-YANG THEORY

Genesis

The yin-yang theory was born in ancient China. This can be seen in *Yi Jing* ("The Book of Changes") written during the Zhou Dynasty (11th century-221 B.C.) in which the relationship between the eight natural matters is explained as the origin of the world: heaven (*qian* ☰), earth (*kun* ☷), thunder (*zhen* ☳), fire (*li* ☲), wind (*xun* ☴), marsh (*dui* ☱), water (*kan* ☵), and mountain (*gen* ☶). Among these eight, heaven and earth are said to be the most basic. In *bagua*[13] (eight trigrams), – stands for yang and – – for yin. The different combinations of these two symbols form a variety of divinatory diagrams representing the different relationships and the overlap between yin and yang, which oppose each other but coexist in a single unity. *Yi Jing* draws this pair of opposites from the complex natural and social world, maintaining that yin and yang make up *dao* (way), or *tao* spelt in the Wade system, in the universe. That is to say that the unity between yin and yang is the law of creation.

The idea that the opposition of yin and yang within things creates constant changes embodies scientific truth. This concept is still significant even in modern and contemporary science. For example, Gottfried Wilhelm Leibniz (1646-1716), the well-known German natural scientist, mathematician and philosopher, spent a dozen years designing and making the forerunner of the computer. He worked out various plans but ultimately failed. One day he received a letter from a missionary friend living in Beijing, China; enclosed was an ancient Chinese picture of *bagua*. He carefully examined the picture and saw the unending changes formed by the different patterns of connections between the symbols of "- -" and "–". This gave him new insight and understanding, from which he went on to create the binary system of "0" and "1". Leibniz had solved the long-standing and difficult problem in the design of computers, and in 1701 succeeded in making the world's first hand-operated computer. The binary system created by Leibniz is still being used in the most advanced and most complicated computers. He himself confessed that the idea for his binary system came from the Chinese picture of *bagua*.

In 1973, Goldberg gained a great deal of insight from *bagua* in a periodical introducing Chinese medicine. Soon afterwards, he presented the well-known "hypothesis of yin and yang" in the human body. He asserted that cAMP (cyclic adenosine monophosphate) and cGMP (cyclic guanine monophosphate) are the two opposing regulatory systems within the human body which form an equilibrium between yin and yang; this hypothesis will be dealt with later in this book. How is this concept of opposition and unity between yin and yang conceived? According to *Yi Jing*, it comes from a look at what is around you or stands far away from you. What is around you refers to man and woman, life and death, up and down, prosperity and decline, while those standing far away from you include natural phenomena such as the sky and the earth, the sun, the moon and the stars, the change of the weather and seasons, as well as some social phenomena such as calamity and happiness, beauty and ugliness, and good and evil. All these phenomena are opposing yet related, and are in constant change and development, and a philosophical conception of the unity between yin and yang is the source of changes and development.

This concept of unity found its way into Chinese medical science in its early stage and became its guiding principle. *Huang Di Nei Jing* ("The Canon of Medicine of the Yellow Emperor"), first Chinese medical classic, appeared during the Qin (221-207 B.C.) and Han (206 B.C.-220 A.D.) dynasties, and claimed, "Yin and yang are *dao* of the universe, the law and order of creation, the father and mother of changes, the beginning of life and death, and the home of man's soul." The unity between yin and yang, as ancient Chinese believed, is the law governing all the things in the world, and the cause of both motion and change and growth and decay. It can also be used to learn about by means of thinking. In both medical theory and clinical practice, the concept of the unity between yin and yang and that of *wuxing*[14] (five elements) is reflected in everything— from nature to the human body, from the part to the whole in organism, from physiology to pathology, from diagnosis to treatment, and from prescription to drug. It is on this basis that Chinese medicine has built its own system. This will be dealt with in the next section of the book.

Integration of Yin and Yang

This concept is reflected in the traditional Chinese outlook on nature; its understanding of the relationship between the human body and nature, physiology and pathology, diagnosis and treat of disease; and its conception of prescriptions and drugs, health protection and the preservation of life.

Outlook on Nature
Chinese medical science has its outlook on nature. The integration of yin and yang is the universal law of things, the source of motion and change, and the origin

of the spiritual world. The earth is in the center of a void. How does it hang? It is held up by the atmosphere.... What is above runs to the right. What is below runs to the left. The movements to the left and right revolve in a cycle[15]. Ancient Chinese physicians realized that the earth hangs in a void in the universe, and that the universe revolves towards the right (from east to west), while the earth revolves towards the left (from west to east). As these two opposites are contradictory to each other, the earth keeps in constant motion.

Traditional Chinese medicine adopts a materialistic point of view on the creation of the universe. *Huang Di Nei Jing* says, "In the vast universe genes and natural energies were created. All things have their beginnings. The movement of *wuxing* is eternal. The universe is in full command of yin and yang. Nine stars are hanging above and shining brightly while seven shining stars (*qi yao*) revolve in their orbits. The process of creating and changing goes on continuously. Everything is complete and in order." This illustrates that the universe is void, vast and spacious. Its origin is due to the creation and changes in natural energy. In the universe, all things mutually attract and respond, working and moving constantly in cycles. Laws govern *wuxing* and *liuqi*. Spring, summer, autumn and winter maintain their own respective schedules. The natural energy of the universe is distributed to everything in the universe: above, the sun, moon and stars move, revolve and shine; below, *qi* grows on earth. All this shows that there is an orderly relationship between yin and yang— of light and dark, cold and heat, day and night— indicating the way things constantly grow and change, and making it possible for them to spread and flourish. This conception reflects the brilliant materialist thought of the ancestors of the Chinese people.

The reason for the motion and change of things in the world is the change in the relationship between yin and yang. According to *Huang Di Nei Jing*, all things may rise or fall and come or go, and for this reason they grow and change. When *qi* decreases, they will fall apart and cease growing and changing. Changes may be great or small, and take place at different times. Yet the most important for things is to keep stable. There is a link between high and low, and rise and fall when changes take place. Yin and yang link with and condition each other, and each is the source of the other. *Huang Di Nei Jing* also says, "Without yin, yang cannot create anything, nor can yin without yang." That is to say that they are conditioning and inseparable; if one of them dies away, the other will not exist any longer and life will disappear. According to *Huang Di Nei Jing*, there is yang in yin and yin in yang. The yang in heaven is just yang of yang from morning till noon and the yin of yang from noon till evening, while the yin in heaven is just yin of yin and the yang of yin from night till daybreak. This shows that yang and yin not only permeate each other but grow or decline together. In the daytime, yang contains yin, but yin will take the place of yang and occupy the dominant position when the former develops and surpasses the latter, and with that, day will turn into night. Likewise, when yin recedes and yang grows, night will turn into day.

Ancient Chinese physicians also had some knowledge about the relationship between quantitative and qualitative changes. According to *Huang Di Nei Jing*, the appearance of a certain thing comes from dissolution but the disappearance of it from transformation; the growth leads to success but the decline to failure. Changes take place when a certain thing is in motion. That is to say that everything is in motion and success or failure depends on motion; when quantitative change reaches a certain level, qualitative change will take place. Dealing with transformation and dissolution separately, as found in *Huang Di Nei Jing*, shows that quantitative and qualitative changes are different and inseparable.

An alternation of excess and deficiency between yin and yang is often mentioned in books on traditional

Chinese medicine. According to *Huang Di Nei Jing*, yin will give rise to yang when it becomes extreme, and vice versa. When the struggle between yin and yang reaches a certain level, a thing will turn into its opposite. That is just the law of the negation of negation.

The above-mentioned points of view can be seen everywhere in many books on traditional Chinese medicine such as *Shang Han Lun* ("Treatise on Febric Diseases Caused by Cold"). It is according to these points of view that the onset, development and changes of febrile disease as well as its prognosis and transmission are explained. Reading that book, you can find that the struggle between yin and yang brings about changes in *liujing*[16] (six channels)— three yang channels and three yin ones formed in the process of febrile disease. Traditional medicine holds the viewpoint of "balance between promotion and inhibition, and the harm of hyperfunction." It claims that if yin and yang and *wuxing* promote and inhibit each other, and the system of a person's life keeps its balance, his body will maintain peace and health; if yin or yang is stimulated too much and its opposite fails in inhibition, the body will lose its balance, placing everything within it out of order, and a certain illness will befall him. Consequently, the balance of generation and inhibition and the harm of hyperfunction is an extremely important guide in traditional clinical practice.

The Relationship Between Man and Nature

According to traditional Chinese medicine, the human body is an organic part of the universe, so that yin and yang in the body and those in nature are closely related and mutually conditioned. For example, changes in the weather and in the seasons have some effect on the production of yin and yang in the human body. *Huang Di Nei Jing* says, "Man is born from the energies of heaven and earth, and his pattern of life is shaped by the law of the four seasons.... Heaven feeds man with *wuqi*[17] (five kinds of *qi*) and earth feeds him with *wuwei*[18] (five kinds of flavor).... He is born when those kinds of *qi* are in harmony, and vitality comes forth spontaneously when life essence and body fluid support each other mutually." The conclusion is that "man is intermingled with heaven and earth and corresponds to the movement of the sun and the moon." This points to the relationship between the body and nature, and that between spirit and matter and *qi* in yin and yang which are mutually creative. These are the material basis that gives birth to vitality. As early as 770-476 B.C., the theory of *liuqi* as causes of disease was recorded in *Zuo Shi Chun Qiu* ("Master Zuo's Spring and Autumn Annals"). This was supported by the famous physician, Doctor He. He said, "Heaven is endowed with *liuqi* that produces *wuwei*, *wuse*[19] (five colors) and *wusheng*[20] (five kinds of sound). *Liuqi*, if excessive, may cause six kinds of illness through wind, cold, damp-heat, dampness, dryness and fire. *Liuqi*, yin, yang, wind, rain, darkness and brightness are distributed among the four seasons and arranged in five stages. If excessive, something unexpected will occur such as too much yin, cold, yang, heat and wind. Too much wind will cause paralysis; too much rain, abdominal disorder; too much darkness, worries; and too much brightness, heart trouble." The concept of inter-penetration and correspondence of human beings with the natural world was later developed into that of *liujing* and *liuqi*, *wuyun* and *liuqi* as well as *ziwuliuzhu* and other theories in traditional Chinese medicine. These will be discussed in the following chapters.

Physiology and Pathology

Human physiology in modern medicine involves the study of processes of the human body and the laws of their functions. These functions involve the physiological processes as well as the systems and organs; the laws are manifested in respiration, circulation, digestion, excretion, reproduction and movements of muscles, etc. Physiology also explains the causes and conditions of these functions, and the effects of the internal and external environment on them. The three levels of human physiology are that of the whole body, of organs and systems, and of cells or molecules, all of which are studied and analyzed on the basis of anatomy.

Pathology in modern medicine is the study of the nature of diseases. Its task is to discover their causes, the part of the body affected, and the body's reactions. It also seeks to learn the changes in the functions, the metabolism, and the laws of transformation during the development of the disease and to recognize the disease's substance. In the past, under the influence of Virchow's cytopathology, the study of patho-anatomy was emphasized, and people spent much time learning about the changes in the structure of the organs, tissues and cells of the affected body and exploring the mechanism of the onset and the changes in the disease.

The body is dissected and analyzed by means of the analytical method prevailing in modern physiology and pathology, with systems and organs coming first and tissues, cells and molecules second. In the mind's eyes of scientists, there is no way of knowing the body as a whole if the local structures of molecules, cells, tissues, organs and systems have not yet learned about. The rapid development of modern science and technology has made it possible for physiologists and pathologists to make a deep study of organs, tissues, cells, molecules and electrons while exploring their secrets, and in so doing, their knowledge of the body increased greatly.

Owing to different social and historical conditions, traditional Chinese medical specialists did not study physiology and pathology in terms of molecules, cells and tissues, but instead of the whole body. They built an orderly understanding of the integration of yin and yang and of the inter-promotion and restraint in the five *zang* organs, and an ideal pattern of their movement and development, in order to construct its own theory of *zang-fu* organs, and guided by this theory, they discovered the physiological and pathological mechanisms in the human body.

Traditional Chinese medicine believes that the human body was first created through the copulation of yin and yang. *Huang Di Nei Jing* says, "Two kinds of *qi* attract each other and mingle into a physical entity.... Yang changes into *qi*, while yin constitutes the entity." *Qi* is yang, while the essence of the body is yin; matter and energy (the physical body and its function) mutually grow and nurture each other. Yang is rooted in yin, and yin in yang. "Without yang, yin cannot give birth; without yin, yang cannot change."

Regarding the structure of the body, *Huang Di Nei Jing* says, "When talking about the yin and yang of man, the exterior is yang, while the interior is yin, the back is yang, while the abdomen is yin. When speaking about *zang-fu* organs, the *zang* ones belong to yin, while the *fu* ones are yang. That is, the heart, liver, spleen, lung and kidney are yin, while the gallbladder, stomach, large intestine, small intestine, bladder and triple energizer are yang. The yang of yang is the heart; the yin of yang is the lung. The abdomen is yin. The yin of yin is the kidney; the yang of yin is the liver; the extreme yin of yin is the spleen. Yin and yang, exterior and interior, female and male are all mutually correspond. This corresponds to the yin and yang in the universe." That is, the relationship between the different parts of the human body and between these parts and the outside environment match that between yin and yang.

The function of *qi* is yang, and the *jing* of the physique is yin. That is that yang changes into *qi* and yin constitutes the entity. According to *Huang Di Nei Jing*, yin preserves the *jing* of life and provides the motive, while yang guards against an invader and unites with the interior. Yin is inside and forms the basis of yang; yang is outside and lays the foundation for yin. The physical entity (yin) and *qi* (yang) grow and nurture each other. *Huang Di Nei Jing* also says that the lucid yang finds its vent through upper apertures, turbid through lower apertures. The lucid yang exits from *couli*, while the turbid yin goes into the five *zang* organs; the lucid yang replenishes the four limbs, while the turbid yin returns to the six *fu* organs. The *qi* of the lucid yang may replenish the skin and nourish the four limbs. The matter of the turbid yin is stored in the five *zang* organs and discharged from the six *fu* organs after undergoing metabolism. The ascent and descent of yin and yang, their outgoing and incoming motion, demonstrate the body's physiological activities.

The concept of the integration of opposites between yin and yang also permeates traditional Chinese thinking regarding health and disease. Details will be discussed in the following chapters; only a general observation will be made here. *Huang Di Nei Jing* says, "If yin is at peace and comfortable, and yang permeates perfectly, one's spirit will be buoyant." That is to say that man will be healthy both physically and mentally if his yin is in a state of balance, and his yang is preserved and without being too much exposed. At the same time, stability within the human body— constituted by the inter-promotion and restraint between yin and yang, and between *wuxing*— is also an indispensable prerequisite for health. If equilibrium is destroyed or impaired and the bodily balance disturbed, then diseases will breed. As *Huang Di Nei Jing* puts it, when there is too much yin, yang will be diseased, and vice versa.... When yang is deficient, exogenic cold will come, but when yin is deficient, endogenic heat will arrive. On the other, too much yang may lead to exogenic heat, but too much yin may give rise to endogenic cold. The development of a disease is a process of struggle— decline and growth and changes— between yin and yang. According to *Huang Di Nei Jing*, when cold goes to its extreme, heat will arrive, but when heat goes to its extreme, cold will come. In other words, a thing turns into its opposite when pushed too far. This point of view can be seen clearly in Zhang Zhongjing's

Shang Han Lun in which the development of febrile diseases is said to be a process of change from three yang channels to three yin ones. Zhang says in his book that when a person has just come down with pathogenic factors (cold, for example), he is quite strong, and the early symptoms are only high fever and ache all over with constipation, owing to diseases in yang channels, but when he is weakened by the disease, some other symptoms will be found such as vomiting, diarrhea, weak pulse, cold extremities and drowsiness, and the reason is that his yang channels have become three yin channels. However, when his resistance becomes stronger, three yin channels will turn into three yang ones and his health be regained. According to *Jin Kui Yao Lue Fang Lun* ("Synopsis of Prescriptions of the Golden Chamber"), also written by Zhang Zhongjing, when the liver is found to be affected, the doctor will prepare a prescription for the spleen instead of the liver because he believes that the liver disease will spread to the spleen. Learn about the relationships between the inter-promotion and restraint of *wuxing* and the five *zang* organs and you will know how to prevent and treat diseases. It is the integration of yin and yang, as Zhang Zhongjing points out in his *Shang Han Lun* and *Jin Kui Yao Lue Fang Lun*, that gives rise to the development and change of diseases.

Diagnosis and Treatment

The principal methods used in Western medicine are based on dissection and analysis of the human body, to discover the location, cause and effect of the disease. Along with examining the symptoms and bodily signs in accordance with the requirements of physiology and pathology, diagnosis emphasizes the physical, chemical and histological means to open the black box and observe the changes taking place in the affected organs, tissues, cells and body fluids; also observed are such pathogenic elements as parasites, bacteria and viruses.

With the development of science and technology,

many new methods have appeared to explore the human body. The electron microscope may help observe pathogenic microbes and even more infinitesimal forms and structures in histiocytes inside the human body. Electronic computer-assisted tomography (CAT) can help know more about the structure of the organs and their changes from different sides and layers. Ultrasonic diagnosis may detect the organic parenchyma inside the body by means of ultrasonic waves. Electrocardiograms, electroencephalography and electromyograms can show the condition of organ functions. All these play a great role in medical diagnosis. A tendency now, however, is that quite a few doctors are depending more and more on physical, chemical and histological examinations in practice.

The therapeutic principle of Western medicine is also used to ascertain the causes of diseases such as those caused by bacteria, virus, rickettsias, spirochete, fungi and parasites, tissue trauma, and loss of equilibrium between internal environmental factors like nerves, body fluid and others in order to find the site of the diseases and apply a corresponding treatment. With this method, the causes of the disease will be eliminated and the pathological process be changed.

Due to the differences in methodology and scientific and technological conditions, four methods are usually adopted in traditional Chinese medicine, namely— observation, ausculation and olfaction, inquiry, pulse feeling and palpation— to explore the symptoms and signs of the diseases. Judging from the information gained, a guiding principle is developed to decide on the nature of a disease. This guiding principle consists of four pairs of categories: exterior and interior, cold and heat, deficiency and excess, and yin and yang. These are also called the "eight principles." Of these eight, yin and yang are regarded as the general guiding principles. Interior, cold and deficiency belong to yin by nature while exterior, heat and excess are yang. Yin and yang are also regarded as guiding principles for the location of the disease— whether in the five *zang* or the six *fu* organs— and the forming of concepts such as *qi* and blood, body fluid, and physique and vitality. And the notion of confrontation, integration, struggle, growth and decline between yin and yang is also used to form a correct diagnosis on a disease and predict its future development.

The final reason of a disease, according to traditional Chinese medicine, is an imbalance between between yin and yang and disorder of *wuxing*, so what should be done first and foremost is to adjust the relationship between them. The heat syndrome should be treated with cold-natured drugs, the cold syndrome with hot-natured drugs, prolapse and ptosis with lifting method, the deficiency syndrome with reinforcing or replenishing method, the excess syndrome with method of purgation and reduction, and so on. All these, along with ascending, descending, floating and sinking (as descriptions of the direction of a drug's movement), treating *qi* or blood, nourishing yin or replenishing yang— aim at "readjusting yin and yang to bring about balance between them and reinforcing *qi* and building up the body's resistance to eliminate the pathogenic factors.

In traditional Chinese medicine, there are eight therapeutic methods: diaphoresis, emesis, purgation, mediation, heat-clearing, warming, resolution and tonification. As ancient Chinese physicians pointed out, diaphoresis is used when the pathogenic factors are outside and yang is prevented from defending the body; emesis used when those factors are at the upper part of the body, and yang are unable to ascend as normal; purgation used when the factors are at the middle or lower region, preventing yang from settling in the middle, or causing constipation and congestion in the lower portion; mediation used when there is discord between exterior and interior, upper and lower, and liver and spleen; the clearing method used when excessive pathogenic heat prevails in the *qi*, nutrient and blood systems but without any outside excess (constipation or obstruction); the warming method used when pathogenic cold in yin invades the *jingluo* system and the *zang-fu* organs; "resolution" used when there is stagnation in *qi* and stasis in blood, sputum-retention, water-stagnation and indigestion-stagnation, and that is to "get rid of the superfluous;" and tonification used when there is no enough *qi* or physical strength, and that is to "replenish something missing." All these methods are created to regulate yin and yang, and restore the part that *wuxing* plays.

The concept of confrontation and integration between yin and yang and that of the sequential influence among the *zang-fu* organs is the fundamental law governing traditional Chinese medicine in the diagnosis and treatment of diseases.

Prescriptions and Drugs

The main task of pharmacology in Western medicine is to analyze the component, chemical composition, and the structure of drugs. It is on this basis that this school of medicine probes shows how the various components act on the human body and its pathogens, along with structural and metabolic changes, so as to prevent and cure disease and protect health. In recent years, progress in physiology and biochemistry has given a stimulus to the further development in the receptor theory of the effect of drugs, which deals with the preventive and curative effect produced by matching the molecular structure of a drug with the structure of certain components in a part of the cell. The principal method used in Western medicine starts with an analysis and then makes an experiment in hopes of opening up as deeply as possible the black box of both drugs and the human body. This method helps Western scientists learn more about the drugs and their effects on the body.

Traditional Chinese medicine, on the contrary, does not deal with the method to open the black box of drugs or the body. Its main job is to discover the nature, taste, function, and the effect of a drug by studying its effect and the body's response to it. To obtain such information requires thousands of repeated practices, comparisons and personal experiences, all of which are summarized and guided by the principle of yin and yang and *wuxing*.

There are various prescriptions in traditional Chinese medicine, and according to their effects they may fall into ten types: obstruction-removing, dispelling, tonifying, purgative, light diaphoretic, heavy, lubricating, astringent, desiccating, and moistening. The first type of prescription is used for stasis or obstruction, the second for stasis, phlegm and emesis, the third for deficiency, the fourth for constipation and excessive heat, accumulated cold and retained body fluid, the fifth for diaphoresis, the sixth for fear, the seventh for dysuria and the discharging of calculi, the eighth for excessive sweat, seminal emission and protracted diarrhea, the ninth for pathogenic dampness, and the tenth for the replenishing of body fluid. All those kinds of prescription are used in terms of yin and yang and *wuxing* according to the law of unity of opposites, and yin and yang should be a guiding principle in determining a prescription's ingredients.

A prescription in Chinese medicine usually consists of four parts, with each having its own effect on the disease. They are *jun* (the principal), *chen* (the adjuvant), *zuo* (the auxiliary) and *shi* (the conductor). As Li Dongyuan (1180-1251), a physician in the Jin Dynasty (1115-1234), put it, a disease has several causes. The main cause should be removed by an ingredient called *jun* but other causes must be dealt with by those belonging to *zuo* and *shi*. That is so important in preparing a prescription. In other words, those ingredients called *jun* are used to treat the main symptom, while those regarded as *chen* are for the enhancing of its effect and those known as *zuo* are for the restraining of the potency of *jun* ingredients when they are too strong or weak. As for *shi* ingredients, they are usually given to help other ingredients with their effects right on the affected part or coordinate the effects of other ingredients.

The above prescription-preparing theory is a law used widely in traditional Chinese medicine. What is most important is to find out the main contradiction, and to treat the main cause of the disease first. That does not mean that you can show any neglect for other causes; instead, you are required to use other ingredients to deal with other causes, and, at the same time, pay attention to coordinating the effects of various ingredients on the disease.

In his book *Ben Cao Bei Yao* ("Essentials of Materia Medica"), Wang Ang (1615-?), a physician living in the early years of the Qing Dynasty (1644-1911), summed up some points about pharmacology prevailing in *Huang Di Nei Jing* and *Ben Cao Gang Mu* ("Compendium of Materia Medica"). He said, "Coldness, hotness, warmness and coolness are *siqi* (the properties of drug), while pungency, sweetness, sour, bitterness and saltness are *wuwei*. *Siqi* belongs to yang, but *wuwei* to yin. When *siqi* is strong, there will be yang in yang, but when *siqi* is less strong, there will be yin in yang; when *wuwei* is thick, there will be yin in yin, but when *wuwei* is less thick, there will be yang in yin. The drug with less strong *siqi* helps you sweat out but that with strong *siqi* makes you hot, while the drug with thick *wuwei* serves as purgatives but that with less thick *wuwei* helps remove obstruction. The pungent and sweet drug with a dissipating effect belongs to yang, but the sour and bitter drug with a draining and purgative effect to yin. The salty drug with a gushing and purgative effect is yin but the thin-flavored drug with a draining and purgative effect is yang. The light and clear things that ascend and float in the body are yang, but the heavy and turbid ones that sink and descend are yin. Yang-*qi* (the properties belonging to yang) runs through the upper orifices, but yin-*wei* (the flavors belonging to yin) goes by way of the lower orifices. The lucid yang evaporates through the skin, but the turbid yin moves through the five *zang* organs; the lucid yang replenishes the four limbs, but the turbid yin assembles in the six *fu* organs. That is what yin and yang implies." Obviously, *siqi* and *wuwei* in materia medica aim to bring about the readjustment of relationship between yin and yang in the human body.

It should be noted, moreover, that the yin and yang in *siqi* and *wuwei* are believed to have something to do with those in in the natural world. Chinese medicine believes that the yin and yang in *siqi* and *wuwei* are related to those in the natural world. Li Dongyuan said, "Drugs may be cold, warm, cool or hot, and their flavors can be pungent, sweet, sour, bitter or salty. Some drugs will be ascending and floating in the body after being taken, but others will be descending and sinking. In addition, there are some other differences between them. Sometimes, the property is the same but the flavor is different, and sometimes the flavor is the same but the property is different. Property may be compared to heaven, and warmness and hotness belong to yang in heaven but coolness and coldness are yin in heaven. Heaven possesses the attributes of yin and yang, wind, cold, summer-heat, dampness, dryness, fire, three yin and three yang channels, all of which reflect the existence of yin and yang in heaven. Flavor is likened to earth, which possesses the attributes of yin, yang, metal, wood, water, fire, earth, creation, growth, change and reaping. Pungent, sweet and plain flavors belong to yang in the earth; sour bitter and salty flavors are of yin. Yin and yang are also reflected in earth. The clear and light things with *siqi* and *wuwei* can become images, and as heaven is their source, they tend to ascend, while those heavy and turbid ones can turn into physiques, and as earth is their source, they tend to descend." For this reason, to treat diseases in the upper part of the body, the drugs with less strong *siqi* and *wuwei* is prescribed more often than not; for diseases in the lower part, the drugs whose property and flavor are usually less strong are often used. That is the basis of Chinese medical theories.

Many kinds of Chinese drug are found to have double function in clinical practice. For example, ginseng (*Radix Ginseng*), helps increase the level of blood sugar, while the root of astragalus membranaceus (*Radix Astragali*) is good for an increase or decrease in blood pressure. That double function, however, cannot be fulfilled through those drugs alone; adjustment to the balance of yin and yang is necessary in accordance with the principle of *bianzhenglunzhi*.

Health Maintenance

There are many works on health maintenance in traditional Chinese medicine, and various methods created by Chinese people including doctors have proved their worth in improving health and prolonging life. The methods are different from one another, but their principle is the same and that is to adjust the balance of yin and yang and get the function of both the *zang-fu* organs coordinated, as explained in *Huang Di Nei Jing*:

> In ancient times those who had learned *dao* acted according to the changes in yin and yang and in harmony with nature, and practiced self-cultivation. They ate moderately, worked and retired at regular times, and always avoided undue exertion. In so doing, they could be in high spirits and good health, and enjoy a long life. For this aim, try to avoid evil wind and drought carefully, preserve vitality with simple mind and stay away from diseases with good spirit. Moreover, pay attention to having a peaceful mind but never to being afraid of anything, to limbering up your body but not to making it tired, and to keeping *qi* flow smoothly. As for daily life, try to enjoy what you eat and wear, and follow the local customs but not to feel envious of those of high status. In such a society, everyone can get his wish true as pleased and all his needs fulfilled. And only in this way can you maintain your vitality and live to 100 years old.

To sum up, the most important is to cultivate moral character. To reach this level, you have to keep your mind calm, concentrate attention on mental activity, act in accordance with the law of nature and adapt yourself to the seasons so that yin and yang within the body will get coordinated with those in nature. In addition, try your best to be moderate in drinking and eating, lead a regular life and work with adequate rest. While following this style of life, take in *jing* and *qi*, do physical exercises and temper your internal organs so that there will be balance between yin and yang and your body will be improved. For instance, *taijiquan* (*taiji* shadow boxing) serves the purpose well. When you do this exercise, the movements should be light, agile, smooth and lively, just like clouds floating in the sky and water in the stream, with your will directing the flow of *qi* and *qi* controlling your body. After that your body will be relaxed and calm naturally. Doing this traditional health-keeping exercise, you will not only get your muscles and bones limbered up but also make your internal organs work more effectively. This exercise is based on the theory of yin and yang and is therefore called *taijiquan*.

Qigong (breathing exercise) had a long history in China, and as it is good for health, this breathing exercise is catching on across the country. Some researchers believe that there is a method called *tuna* (exhalation and inhalation) in *qigong*, which may help remove obstruction in the *jingluo* system, regulate the flow of *qi* and blood, and acquire balance between yin and yang. The reason is that the vegetative nervous system can be regulated in the process. As you know, the *zang-fu* organs are so important in the human body, and yet they are stimulated and regulated by the vegetative nervous system, which does not move at will like the motor nerves. Because of its autonomy in activity, the vegetative nervous system is also called the autonomic nervous system. This nervous system consists of two smaller systems: sympathetic and parasympathetic, whose functions are different but mutually regulative. Once the sympathetic nervous system is excited, the force within the organs will be mobilized and any changes in the surrounding environment be dealt with. Its function is quite similar to yang in traditional Chinese medicine. On the other side of the picture, when the parasympathetic nervous system is excited, digestion will be promoted, consumption be reduced and energy preserved. That sounds like yin in Chinese medicine. When you do *qigong*, try to breathe with the mind concentrating on *dantian*, a region three centimeters below the navel. The exhaling process will react on the apneustic center and the parasympathetic nervous system is excited, while the inhaling process enhances the excitation of the sympathetic nerves. *Tuna* in *qigong* is such a kind of exercise in which the mind is used to direct the flow of *qi* when you are calm and relaxed all over, and the sympathetic and parasympathetic nervous systems are placed in a state of balance between yin and yang, which is good for health. With this theory as their guiding principle, doctors at the Shanghai Qigong Research Institute have tried to treat high blood pressure by means of *qigong* and gained good results. Of course, *qigong* may also help the lungs improve other bodily functions, causing a large rise and fall in the muscles of the diaphragm which plays the same part as massage treatment in the improvement of the function of the internal organs, facilitating the flow of *qi* and blood, and bringing about changes in internal secretions, which is advantageous to health. *Qigong*, which is also based on the theory of yin and yang, has done much to health maintenance and medical treatment.

Judging from the above explanation, we can find that traditional Chinese medicine has a complete set of theories on physiology, pathology, diagnosis, prescription, medication and health maintenance, which, though rich and varied in content, has much to do with the theory of yin and yang. Armed with this theory people are trying to find the law governing the changing, intricate and complex physiological and pathological phenomena within the human body.

The *Wuxing* Theory and the Order in the Human Body

Ancient Greek materialist philosophers took water or fire as the origin of the world. Ancient Indian philosophers believed that the world originated from earth, water, wind and fire. Ancient Chinese philosophers, however, took matter for the origin of the world. They maintained that it consisted of wood, fire, earth, metal and water, which can be seen very often in human life and labor. These, they believed, were mutually related, conditioned and interchangeable, and could at the same time turn into an orderly control system. It was on this basis that the theory of *wuxing* was developed and became full of naive materialism.

Ancients recognized that the many varieties of matter possessed a certain dynamic generality of the same category (like the isomorphic system in the isomorphic theory of systematics). They drew an analogy between things in the world and made an induction from it, so the five kinds of matter in *wuxing*— wood, fire, earth, metal and water— were said to be a general outline to explain the various things in the world. According to *Shang Shu*, one of the classical books on Confucianism written in the Zhou Dynasty, water moistens what is under, fire burns what is above, wood straightens what is bent, metal transforms and cuts, and earth engages in sowing and reaping. Those that moisten, penetrate downwards, clear and cool belong to "water," those that burn, warm, flare up and hyperfunction to "fire," those that generate, masculinize, harmonize and adapt to changes to "wood"; those that are solemn, solid, tenacious and pure to "metal," and those that nourish, develop and grow to "earth." This method is what distinguishes traditional Chinese medicine from Western medicine. Certain chapters in *Huang Di Nei Jing* note that the things commonly seen in the natural world and in the *zang-fu* organs, along with their functions, have been classified under *wuxing*, as shown in the following diagram:

	Wuxing				
	Wood	**Fire**	**Earth**	**Metal**	**Water**
Human Body					
Zang Organs	Liver	Heart	Spleen	Lung	Kidney
Fu Organs	Gall Bladder	Small Intestine	Stomach	Large Intestine	Urinary Bladder
Five Sense Organs	Eyes	Tongue	Mouth	Nose	Ears
Configuration and Constitution	Muscle	Arteries and Veins	Flesh	Skin and Hair	Bone
Emotions	Anger	Joy	Anxiety	Grief	Appreciaciation
Wusheng	Shouting	Laughing	Singing	Wailing	Groaning
Changes	Detention	Stagnation Obstruction	Hiccup and Retching	Expectorating	Shivering
Natural World					
Season	Spring	Summer	Long Summer	Autumn	Winter
Process of Development	Beginning of Life	Growth	Dissolution	Reaping	Storing
Climate	Wind	Summer Heat	Dampness	Dryness	Cold
Wuse	Blue	Red	Yellow	White	Black
Wuwei	Sour	Bitter	Sweet	Pungent	Salty
Wuyin	*Jue*	*Zhi*	*Gong*	*Shang*	*Yu*

That testifies to the fact that the *zang* organs correspond to *wuxing* with the liver being of the wood genus, the heart of fire, the spleen of earth, the lung of metal, and the kidney of water. This is because they have similar attributes and features. For instance, the liver produces and transforms nutrients inside the body and needs nourishment from the body fluid and blood of the kidney, just as wood needs comfort, ease and flexibility. The heart beats constantly, like the flames of a fire. It injects and lets red blood flow and produces heat energy. Since these are the specific properties of fire, the heart is believed to be of the fire genus. The function of the spleen is similar to that of the earth, which is the home of many things, since it can digest and absorb nutrients for the organism and is the foundation of postnatal cultivation. The lung is like metal: it is effected by the air (as in breathing and oxidation) and makes sounds when vibrating. The kidney possesses specific properties similar to those of water, with a tendency to flow down and discharge. It nourishes and moistens the *zang-fu* organs, and when energizing (somewhat like evaporating), it moistens the whole body. The concept of analyzing the relationship between the *zang-fu* organs on the one hand and between *wuwei*, *wuse* and *wusheng* in the natural world and *wuxing* on the other, has been widely applied in traditional Chinese medical theory and clinical practice.

The methods— comparing similarities to seek identical and using samples to draw analogies— were customarily used in the theory of *wuxing* in Chinese medicine. These methods analyze and classify the qualities and special features of things in the same category. An organic relationship between them is then established through comparison and analogy. These two methods are frequently mentioned in *Huang Di Nei Jing*, which says, "You will feel confused if you don't know how to discriminate between the different categories of medicine." These methods of analogical thinking are based on the materialist principle of the diversity and unity of matter. Although the relationship between different kinds of matter can be learned about according to this principle, the conclusion to which it leads is only a probability, still, it might help in formulating ideas through creative thinking. Ancient Chinese physicians demonstrated creative thinking in medical science, which was used to guide their clinical practice. They could even foresee certain medical ideas which have become known only recently. In the history of science, there have been many precedents for original creative ideas through analogical association. When August Kekule von Stradonitz (1829-1896), the famous German chemist, was studying the structure of the organic chemical benzene, he imagined the atom to be a cluster of snakes snapping at each other's tails. Enlightened by this association, he presented the world-famous theory of the ring structure of the benzene molecule, composed of six carbon atoms and six hydrogen atoms.

The most important point in the theory of *wuxing* is its concept of generation, inhibition, encroachment and overpowering; this is because it embodies spontaneous dialectic thinking. The so-called inter-generation of *wuxing* claims that wood generates fire, fire generates earth, earth generates metal, metal generates water and water generates wood; while according to inter-inhibition, wood inhibits earth, earth water, water fire, fire metal and metal wood. In the relationship of inter-generation, each element consists of two phases: "generating" and "generated," which are likened to the relationship between ''dominating" and "dominated," and are in turn similar to that between the mother and her son in *Nan Jing* ("On Difficult Medical Problems"). In the relationship of inter-inhibition, each also consists of two phases, which are "dominating" and "dominated" in *Huang Di Nei Jing*. In the relationship between generation and inhibition, generation signifies birth and growth of matter, and inhibition the mutual conditioning of opposites. Generation and inhibition show that things are connected, conditioned and interchangeable; they mutually generate and mutually inhibit, mutually oppose and mutually complement; they advance the movement and development of material growth and decline. If one element of *wuxing* is too oppressive, a corresponding element will inhibit it so that there is balance between yin and yang, just like feedback regulation in modern science. *Huang Di Nei Jing* states: "Utmost dominance will result in a recovery; after the recovery, dominance will be regained. Harm will ensue if there is no recovery." This explains the cause very well. Consequently, mutual generation and mutual inhibition signify the normal relationship between all the elements of *wuxing*. The so-called "encroachment" refers to invasion through a vulnerable spot. Thus, if liver-wood is excessively dominant, it will seek a vulnerable spot in spleen-earth whereby wood inhibits earth, and the spleen becomes sick. Overpowering means the coercion of the weaker by the stronger. For instance, while metal normally inhibits wood, excessively dominant liver-wood overpowers metal, causing lung-metal to become sick. Encroachment and overpowering therefore signify a disturbance in the normal harmonious relationship between things due to a hyperfunction or hypofunction that gives rise to diseases. *Huang Di Nei Jing* says, "Hyperfunction causes harm and should be checked. When it is checked, generation and metamorphosis prevail, and thriving or declining appears on the outside. Harm courts defection and disorder to the detriment of generation and metamorphosis." According to Zhang Jingyue (1563-1640), author of several books on special subjects such as gynecology, pediatrics and surgery, the mechanism of generation and metamorphosis will not work without generation or inhibition. Without generation, there will be no ground for growth and development; without inhibition, hyperfunction will ensue and cause harm. In other words, too much growth and development (hyperfunction) are harmful; only when things condition one another can they maintain a relative balance, which is good to both generation and metamorphoses.

A model pattern of generation, inhibition, conditioning and metamorphosis of the body on the basis of the theory of *wuxing* may be like the following map. The relatively stable mechanism between the five *zang* organs maintained through the various feedback circuits is much like the cybernetic theory of the homeostasis.

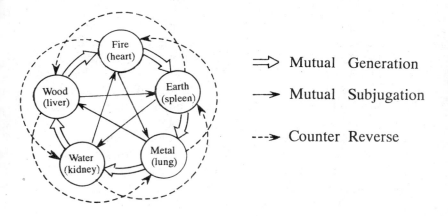

In their article *Chinese Medicine— A Miracle in the History of Sciences*, Hua Guofan and Jin Guantao said:

> The homeostasis, otherwise called the super stabilized system, was first mentioned by Aishibi, the well-known expert in cybernetics. In his book *Design of the Cerebrum*, he described in detail the special features of this apparatus, characterized by its imitation of a structurally complex system capable of automatically maintaining stability. As is shown in the diagram, the homeostasis is composed of A, B, C, D and E— five subsystems of mutual feedback relations.
>
> The homeostasis possesses two interesting features: First, if one section of the system (for instance, subsystem A) deviates somewhat from the state of equilibrium, the reaction of the other subsystems will help to restore it. But if the deviation is sufficiently

large, and the reaction of the subsystems is unable to help subsystem A restore its equilibrium within a short time, then ... one or several other subsystems may also deviate. Second, if there is only one equilibrium in the system, then irrespective of its initial state, it will eventually regain stability through interaction between the various subsystems. As long as the system is unstable, it will continuously seek equilibrium.

These two important properties of the homeostasis are widespread in the human body. If the A, B, C, D and E subsystems in the diagram are taken for each element of *wuxing* or each of the five *zang* organs, and the basic stability of the system is the health of a normal human body, then the pathological state is the outcome of a disease in the homeostasis. The control technology built on the basis of the theory of *zang-fu* organs actually utilizes the external input to the diseased state and restore it to health.

The concept of stability in the theory of *zangxiang* is very basic. The variables of the different systems within the *zang* organs show a relationship between mutual nourishment, generation and mutual promotion. Others manifest the progressively decreasing relationship of mutual conditioning and restriction. They constitute a complex regulating relationship interwoven with various kinds of positive and negative feedback circuits. There is conditioning in the generation and there is generation in the conditioning; they are both opposite and complementary to each other and operate by themselves continuously, whereby the various movements of life and the various functions in the body maintain a relative stability. Under normal conditions, such a stability is strongly maintained. The organism might have been repeatedly disturbed by various external factors, and the equilibrium might even have been in a state of constant fluctuation. Because each internal organ has its own disease-resistant power, and there is a mechanism of mutual coordination between the various visceral systems, the changes may not easily be able to surpass a certain threshold value. Therefore, the basic variables of the various visceral systems are able to maintain relative stability.... However, if internal and external pathogenic factors are too strong and the state of certain *zang* organs is forced to surpass the relative equilibrium needed to preserve health, the body will be affected by diseases. The model pattern of the *zang-fu* organs provides us with a formula for the transmission of pathogenic disturbances as well as a formula for the coordination of the various energies within the body. Accordingly, we can effectively guide the regulation and control of many diseases by observing this pattern.

The theory of yin and yang and that of *wuxing* maintain that the relationship between things, between the *zang* organs in the body, and between the body and nature has acquired relative equilibrium and stability through the constant inheritance, conditioning, generation and inhibition. There is an orderly and regular holistic relationship as well as one of mutual conditioning. These coincide with the concept of equilibrium and order in modern biology and medicine. People now recognize that the mechanism of living things strictly follow the law of relative equilibrium and order in order to keep a kind of relative stability on which the inside of the mechanism depends for its existence. In the DNA-RNA-protein formation, purine, pyrimidine and various kinds of amino acids are compounded into a nucleotide and a protein, strictly in accordance with a certain composition, array-combination and structural pattern. The structure and activity of the cells are characterized by a material foundation composed of complicated compounds and many kinds of macromolecules, and their assimilation and alienation move in strict accordance with a certain interrelationship and order. Organs are not independent kingdoms administering their own ways, but instead carry out the physiological activities of the whole body in union through extremely complicated and delicate interrelations and in accordance with interactions governed by various laws. But they are all under the control of nerves and body fluid. Excitation and inhibition, feedback and regulation, for instance, are carried on strictly in accordance with the principle of equilibrium and order. Once this is interfered with or destroyed by physical, chemical, biological or mental causes, diseases or even death will ensue if the organism is unable to overcome the chaos. Cancer, for instance, is a process of proliferation in the DNA-RNA-protein and in the cell, which is off the right track when the cell becomes cancerized. The cancer cells distend and proliferate, seriously disturbing the equilibrium and order within the mechanism and finally eating the patient's life away.

Ecological equilibrium and order should also be maintained between living things and the environment; otherwise living things will not be able to exist on the earth. Take some living things in ancient times for example. They became extinct because a great change in the environment destroyed the original ecological equilibrium. These problems have been dealt with in traditional Chinese medicine through the relative equilibrium between yin and yang, and the order of generation, inhibition, conditioning and metamorphosis of *wuxing*, but not enough for some historical reasons. Nevertheless, the dialectic thought contained in it has reflected the wisdom of the Chinese people.

The concept of *wuxing* has been widely applied in clinical practice with good results. *Nan Jing* says, "He who diagnoses by observing the complexion should look for *wuse* of the face to tell the gravity of illness; he who diagnoses by auscultation and olfaction should listen for *wusheng* to differentiate the illness; and he who diagnoses by inquiry should ask the patient which flavor of *wuwei* he likes best, with a view to knowing how the illness originated and where it is located." This makes use of the relationship between the *zang* organs, *wuse, wusheng* and *wuwei* to help diagnose an illness. The book also says, "In the case of an insubstantial syndrome, tonify the maternal viscus; in the case of an excessive syndrome, discharge the filial viscus." This is a therapeutic principle ascertained by applying the relationship of generation and inhibition among *wuxing*. According to *Jin Kui Yao Lue Fang Lun*, to cure a disease before its onset means that when the liver is affected, a prescription is prepared to tonify the spleen, since the doctor knows the liver disease will go into the spleen.... For liver diseases, the drug which is sour should be used to tonify the deficient liver." That tells us that we can make use of the generation and inhibition of *wuxing* and their relationships with *wuwei* to prevent and cure diseases.

It is noteworthy that the theory of *wuxing* reduces the origin of matter to concrete properties. It confuses the philosophical category of matter with its substantial properties, so the infinite diversity in the objective world and the complicated relationship that exists between things cannot be explained in a scientific way. This has been a common defect of ancient naive materialism. Moreover, in terms of methodology, the deduction that results from "comparing similarities to seek identical" is only a probability, not a certainty. It must instead pass through the examination of serious practice; after discarding the dross and selecting the essentials, it can penetrate even deeper to master the innate essence and internal relationships of matter. The rationality of the theory of *wuxing* lies in that it has recognized the materiality of the world and comprehended the antithesis and unity of the contradictions within matter and its processes, as well as the interrelation, interconditioning and interchangeableness— i.e., the internal generation, inhibition, conditioning and metamorphosis of matter— which advances its sequential movement and development. If one departs from these principles and attempts far-fetched analogies that reduce complex natural relations to those merely of *wuxing*, he will limit or distort the reality of matter. In short, we encourage an acceptance of the methods of the traditional Chinese legacy but only after they have been further investigated. We advocate making a thorough study of the theory of *wuxing* in order to assimilate its essence, not its dross. We should also guard against inflexibility and blind acceptance of the theory.

Interrelation Between Nature and Mankind in the Yin-Yang Theory

Engels pointed out that life is the existence of protein, and the basic element of this form of existence is that it constantly metabolizes the external natural world surrounding it; once this ceases, life ceases immediately and protein dissolves. The activity of life and its environment are thus very closely related.

The theory of yin and yang embodies the mutual relationship, interference and correspondence between nature and mankind. Some of these have been mentioned in previous sections; we now intend to inquire into the relationship between yin and yang of the body and that of day and night, as well as of the four seasons.

In the yin-yang theory, importance has been given to the influence that the sun exerts on all things, including human being. Take the twenty-four solar terms for example. It started to be used in farming by the Qin Dynasty, which shows that our ancestors had learned about the movements of the sun and the earth. In the Northern Hemisphere, the day of *Dongzhi* (the Winter Solstice) is the shortest in the year but that of *Xiazhi* (the Summer Solstice) the longest. The length of the day of *Chunfen* (the Spring Equinox) and that of *Qiufen* (the Autumn Equinox) are the same. As our ancestors said, yin is generated by the time of *Xiazhi*, and the day becomes shorter, but yang is generated by the time of *Dongzhi*, and thus the day becomes longer. That is to say that the movement of the position of light from the sun causes the change of the seasons and the decline and growth of yin. According to *Huang Di Nei Jing*, the heaven is yang; the earth, yin, the sun, yang and the moon, yin. Their movement is in order and in conformity with the law. Following the annual alternation of the seasons, living organisms give birth in spring, grow in summer, reap in autumn and hibernate in winter. As ancient Chinese believed, the spring and the summer are yang, during which the living organism flourishes; but the autumn and the winter are yin, during which the pace of life slows and hibernation begins. During the daytime, the sun shines over the earth, and the plants thrive, and photosynthesis can go with carbon dioxide inhaled and oxygen exhaled and rich carbohydrates, protein, fats and other substances are produced; animals are also lively in the daytime, moving around to find their food. When night falls the earth becomes calm; plants begin breathing in oxygen, breathing out carbon dioxide so as to store nutritious materials, while most animals rest to restore their physical strength. That is why our ancestors took the daytime as yang and night as yin. Modern scientists are very interested in studying the "biological clock" that apparently exists within living things. It seems that this is based on the regular influence and action exerted on every living organism by the four seasons and the alternation of day and night, all centering on the sun. Traditional Chinese medicine has paid great attention to the influence of yin and yang of the moon and the sun on those within the body.

Theory holds that *liujing* and *liuqi* are closely related. *Liujing* has much to do with the rising and setting of the sun, seasonal changes and the alternation of yin and yang, while *liuqi* is in relation to seasonal changes brought about by the earth's movement around the sun. In spring people are liable to the wind, which affects the liver and the lung; in summer they are liable to heat, affecting the heart, and they are also liable to dampness, which involves the spleen and the stomach, if the season is quite long; in autumn they are liable to dryness, which affects the lung; and in winter they are liable to cold, affecting the Bladder Channel of Foot-*Taiyang*. According to pulse lore, the pulse is somewhat tight in spring, full in summer, hairy in autumn and stony in winter. These are quite normal, but they may be different with the change of seasons.

The *jingluo* system in traditional Chinese medicine claims that the three yang channels go along the back and the two sides of the body, as well as the dorsal side of the limbs but the three yin channels run along the chest and the abdominal region and the ventral side of the limbs. The *Du* channel, the superintendent of all the yang channels, runs along the midline of the back, facing the sun, while the *Ren* channel, the general director of all the yin channels, along with the midline of the abdomen, facing the shade. The breast and the abdomen are yin and the back is yang, just like our ancestors who crawled on all fours so that they could enjoy sunlight very easily. The *fu* organs netted by these yang channels are those for digestion, absorption and discharge, whose function is very exuberant; this resembles the wigs and leaves of plants, which face the sun and produce nutritious food. Consequently, Chinese medicine maintains that the *fu* organs are attributes of yang. On the other hand, the chest, abdominal region and ventral side of the four limbs are all on the back. The channels going through these parts of the body belong to yin, and the *zang* organs netted by them are used to keep essence of life, like plants whose roots penetrate deeply into the soil to keep their essence and support the trunk. We can see from the above explanations that both theories on the *jingluo* system and *zang-fu* organs have such a point of view that the human body and the sun have much to do with each other.

The *jingluo* theory offers a peculiar understanding of the law of *ziwuliuzhu*, which maintains that the circulation of *qi* and blood in the twelve channels of the body have their peaks and ebbs in a twenty-four hour cycle. The climax hours of *jingluo* is as follows.

The Gallbladder Channel of Foot-*Shaoyang* 23:00-1:00,
The Liver Channel of Foot-*Jueyin* 1:00-3:00,
The Lung Channel of Hand-*Taiyin* 3:00-5:00,
The Large Intestine Channel of Hand-*Yangming* 5:00-7:00,
The Stomach Channel of Foot-*Yangming* 7:00-9:00,
The Spleen Channel of Foot-*Taiyin* 9:00-11:00,
The Heart Channel of Hand-*Shaoyin* 11:00-13:00
The Small Intestine Channel of Hand-*Taiyang* 13:00-15:00
The Bladder Channel of Foot-*Taiyang* 15:00-17:00
The Kidney Channel of Foot-*Shaoyin* 17:00-19:00
The Pericardium Channel of Hand-*Jueyin* 19:00-21:00
The Trio-Jiao Channel of Hand-*Shaoyang* 21:00-23:00

When these channels are in their prime, the essential substances circulating in them become even more vigorous. The theory of *ziwuliuzhu* maintains that the flow of *qi* in the channels has something to do with both the above divisions of time and the year, month and day. If acupuncture, medication or massage is given or *qigong* is practiced when the related channels and foci are open, the effect would be even more pronounced. When a man comes down with a cough or asthma, for example, he will feel too bad; if he is given acupuncture at the *shaoshang* point between 3:00 and 5:00 o'clock in the morning, he will feel much better.

Qigong practitioners advocate doing the exercises early in the morning between 3:00-5:00 a.m., because the lung flourishes during those hours and is in command of *qi* of the whole body; exercise will then achieve the optimum effect. Recent scientific research has also discovered the "around-the-clock regularity of the secretion of a hormone." For instance, secretion of the adrenocortical hormone reaches its peak early in the morning before awakening. This hormone regulates the metabolic equilibrium of water and electrolytes in the body, and coordinates with adrenalin to mobilize sources of *qi* so that the organism can more efficiently adapt to its surroundings. The theory of *ziwuliuzhu* accordingly reflects certain regularities in its exploration of the mutual relationship between the body and the sun, and is worthy of further study and investigation.

There is a special point of view about the rising and setting of the sun and the effects the alternation of the seasons had on disease in traditional Chinese medicine. For instance, *Huang Di Nei Jing* teaches: "Most patients feel sober in the morning, easy in the day, aggravated by the evening and worse during the night." This is because *qi* starts to rise in the morning when illness is weak. As Zhang Zhongjing puts it in his *Shang Han Lun*, there is a fixed time for the alleviation of channel disorder, with the weakening of diseases in the three yang channels happening during the daytime when the yang-*qi* flourishes and that in the three yin channels at night when yin-*qi* is vigorous. One of the obvious disorders in the Stomach Channel of Foot-*Yangming* is tidal fever in the afternoon. That is, the heat of febrile disease or the Stomach Channel of Foot-*Yangming* rises when the sun starts to set, as if it were the beginning of a tide. By night it falls, as if the tide were receding because it is coincident with the time of the flow and ebb of *qi* and blood. The process of development of acute febrile diseases is divided into four stages: *wei* (the superficial defense), *qi*, *ying* (nutrient or constructive) and *xue* (blood)[21]. *Wei* and *qi* belong to yang, for the invasion of the disease is superficial and *qi* within the body is strong and capable of resisting it. *Ying* and *xue* are yin, for the invasion has a harmful effect on the nutrient and blood and has entered a serious stage. When the disease is in the stages of *wei* and *qi*, the disorder is more serious during the daytime than at night, but when it has entered *ying* and *xue* stages, it is more serious at night and the patient's temperature will rise. Chinese medicine maintains that the daytime is yang; yang diseases will consequently be more serious. The night, on the other hand, is yin, and thus yin diseases will be more serious at night. Patients with yang diseases usually perspire in the daytime, but those with yin diseases during the night. Other similar phenomena are seen in clinical practice.

The sun is the fundamental source of energy for the earth, and exercises great influence on all things, including human physiology and pathology. Natural phenomena reveal this to us. The sunflower turns its head towards the sun; woody plants like the silk tree and mimosa extend their leaves towards the sunshine in the morning and roll them up at sunset; flowers like cordate telosma and touch-me-not only give off their sweet scents in the evening; plants photosynthesize in the daytime but perform respiration at night. These examples illustrate the great effect the sun has on the plant physiology.

Animals are beings capable of behaving on their own accord, and their adaptability to the environment is stronger than that of plants. There are also poikilotherms which must hibernate during the cold winter and awake only when spring returns. Some birds such as wild geese fly from the north to the south when autumn comes but return in spring. They are called "climatic" birds (migratory birds) because of their ability to recognize seasonal changes in climate. The pupil of a cat's eye changes shape during the day, resembling a biological clock.. A proverb says about it: "Like a thread during the hours of *zi, wu, mao* and *you*; like a date's pit during the hours of *chen, si, chou* and *wei*; and like a round moon during the hours of *yin, shen, xu* and *hai*[22]." Cat's eyes resemble in their function a biological clock.

The lunar cycle also affects the genital glands of animals. The moon is full during the middle of the lunar month, and at this same time, the ovary and digestive glands of crabs become rich and plump and the clam grows quickly because of increased secretion. Things are different at the beginning of the lunar month when the moon is not full. In his great work *Ben Cao Gang Mu*, Li Shizhen says that the yolk in their belly waxes and wanes like the moon during a crab's reproductive season.

The rooster always crows to announce the arrival of the dawn. How can it keep time so perfectly? Japanese scientists have discovered that its "biological clock" is located in their brain, in the cells of the pineal gland. These cells secrete a hormone called "tensile melanin," which controls the activities of birds. If a capsule full of tensile melanin is placed in the body of a rooster, it will fall asleep. The pineal gland thus functions like a biological clock, remembering the regular alternation of the light and dark. According to the research of American scientists, if a sparrow's pineal gland is removed, it will lose the regularity of the around-the-clock activities; if the gland from another sparrow is transplanted into it, this regularity will be restored. The pineal gland arouses sensitivity to the sunlight because birds can sense the wavelength of light which penetrates their skulls. Light promotes changes inside and outside the cell membrane of the gland and induces a chemical reaction which performs the function of a pendulum in this biological clock.

Inter-continental flights are now increasing, and flying from one time zone to another creates problems due to the time difference. When people enter the new time zone, they feel tired because their biological clock is still running the old time one. In hopes of eliminating this reaction, scientists are studying a kind of medicine that uses the neurohormone secreted by the pineal gland; this would be taken before flying across time zones to accelerate the re-synchronizing action of the biological clock within the human body.

Man's ability to adapt to his environment is greater than any other living things. Because mankind has gradually evolved from the lowest grade of living things, its biological traits are still in the body. That is clear in the development of a fetus, which repeats the different stages of evolution during its growth.

The influence of the sun on human physiology and pathology is certainly real. Cytology shows that the regular activity of choleresis in the liver cells, beneficial for digestion and absorption, predominates during the daytime. Glycogen synthesis in the liver predominates at night, and is beneficial for storing energy. Other parts of the body could also be cited. It is not yet known if a change takes place during the daytime and at night in the circulation of body fluids, the secretion of the endocrine glands and the excitability of vegetative nerves. According to China's *People's Daily* on December 31, 1980, Soviet physicians found that a biological regularity strictly controls the waxing and waning of vitality during the daytime and at night. This regularity helps to determine the dosage of a drug and the time it is to be administered. When vitality and physical strength are in their prime, the body actively consumes energy, and at that time can effectively fight diseases without any help from drug. It is wise, though, to take drug when the body's physiological activities are in a decreased state. Clinical practice has proven that the body's sensitivity to drug is different at different times of the day. Vitamin C is taken before going to bed, results will be best. Patients afflicted with cardiac disease who take digitalis at dawn will find their sensitivity to the medication much greater. Diabetics are also more sensitive to insulin at dawn. Consequently, a new theory called "time therapy" is growing in modern medicine.

Statistics indicate that when yin is declining in strength and yang is rising at dawn, the number of births and deaths is the greatest. Yang is in its prime at noon; if an injury is incurred at that time, blood is most likely to flow, and bleeding will be difficult to stop. People living by the sea often say that bleeding caused by an injury is related to the tidal flow and ebb and that it is usually more copious during flood tide. Physiological functions, such as the secretion cycle of the genital glands, are also related to the waxing and waning of the moon.

An American scientist who has made a study of the influence of the moon on human behavior said that those who have mental disorders are found to have the worst behavior during a full moon. He added that the lunar cycle also has a significant influence on alcoholics and drug addicts. The moon's influence on human psychology is rather complicated. Some scientists maintain that all nerve cells have a small magnetic field. Under ordinary conditions, the magnetic force inside and outside the human body maintains a dynamic balance. When changes take place in the gravitational force and the electric field, they affect the harmony between the body and the world. Such changes make some people angry, nervous, and upset.

Scientists have proved that living things are influenced by the rising and setting of the sun, the alternation of the seasons, and climatic and astronomical changes. For instance, there seems to be a close relationship between sunspots, which occur in 11-year cycles, and the prevalence of influenza. Sunspots release a large quantity of charged particles which creates disturbances in the magnetic field of the earth, causing magnetic explosions. The bio-electric current in the body also creates a small magnetic field, whose magnetic explosions disturb the physiological and pathological activities. Sunspots also affect other things in the natural world, such as animals, plants, the climate and the hydrological situation, and the ecological environment they create also affects the human body. The influenza virus is directly disturbed by these magnetic explosions. A virus can only grow and propagate within living cells. The inherited and duplicated materials inside the virus, DNA or RNA, may become disturbed and relocate in a new subgroup, which the body's immune system may have never encountered before. As a result, this new type of influenza virus affects people more quickly than ordinary types and spreads more rapidly.

If sunspots affect the human body, then other astronomical changes might also have an affect upon the body more or less. *Huang Di Nei Jing* says that attention is paid to the influence exerted on the body by changes of the day, night, seasons, wind, rain, dimness and brightness, as well as astronomical changes. The final conclusion reached is that there is a relationship of mutual affect and response between yin and yang in the natural world and those in the human body. In this field, traditional Chinese medicine has accumulated a great deal of knowledge, expressed in medical theory, therapeutic method, prescription and medicament.

Study of the Yin-Yang Theory in Modern Medicine

The theory of yin and yang is involved in more than methodology, it also comprises theories of physiology, pathology and therapeutic prescription and medicament. Using modern science and technology to explore this theory for the clarification of its basis and principles will be of great significance in the development of traditional Chinese medicine. It will also enrich modern medicine by adding new information and devising new treating methods. Medical workers in China and abroad have become very interested in this field and done much work about it, which should account for quite a few discoveries. This demonstrates that yin and yang are not vague conceptions, but instead real substances within the cells, tissues and organs and that they can be ascertained by means of scientific experiments.

According to an article published in the Shanghai-based *New Medicine and Pharmacy Journal* in 1977, an experiment was made with white mice, and a large dose of acetic hydrate of cortisone was injected into them to bring about exhaustion, a state similar to the deficiency of yang. Their reactions were weight loss, arched back, little activity, slow response, lusterless hairs and an increase in death rate. Changes also took place in their internal organs, such as the swelling of the hepatic cells, decreased nucleic acid, a drop in activities of the succinic acid dehydrogenase, increased glycogen, and decreased Kupffer's cells in the liver; the spleen shrank and a decrease in nucleic aid in the lymphocytes also occurred.

A kind of drug supporting yang consists of *Radix Aconiti*, *Cortex Cinnamomi*, *Herba Cistanchis* and *Herba Epimedii* is likely to improve the deficiency of yang of an organism caused by acetic hydrate of cortisone. After this drug is administered, the nucleic acid content in splenocytes and hepatic cells increases, the activity of succinic acid dehydrogenase increase, glycogen in the spleen decreases and the Kupffer's cells in the liver and lymphocytes in the spleen are protected. It is possible that the aphrodisiac drug first regulates the metabolism of the nucleic acid and, through it, the metabolism of the whole body. The drug increases the succinic acid dehydrogenase, enhances the function of proteins, fats and sugar in the channels to supply the tricarboxylic acid cycle with energy, and increases the content of adenosine triphosphate to reinforce the vitality of the organism.

The deficiency of yin appeared in the mice six days after they were given thyroxin and reserpine— weight loss, increased fidgetiness and uneasiness, a drop in the pain threshold and increased nucleic acid synthesis in the liver and spleen cells. On the eighth and tenth days, the mice became leaner, smaller, and slower in action. The nucleic acid synthesis drops in both the hepatic cells and the hepatic glycogen. This looks somewhat like severe damage of yin and yang that developed into the deficiency of both yin and yang.

If a yin-nourishing decoction compounded with 24 grams each of *Radix Rehmanniae*, *Radix Ophiopogonis* and *Radix Scrophulariae* and 48 grams of *Plastrum Testudinis* is administered to the animals suffering from the deficiency of yin, they will feel better. At the initial stage when nucleic acid synthesis in hepatosplenoid cells increases, this decoction may help decrease it, but when both the deficiency of both yin and yang appears and the nucleic acid synthesis in hepatic cells decreases, this decoction may help it increase. Moreover, it can also increase hepatic glycogen and raise the pain threshold.

Clinical statistics show that the deficiency of yin has something to do with dysthyoidism. When thyroidism occurs, the basal metabolic rate increases, body weight drops, the patient becomes fidgety and uneasy, and there are signs of hyperfunction, like the rise in nucleic acid synthesis and a drop in the pain threshold. The protracted deficiency of yin will result in severe damage of yin. If yang is involved, both yin and yang become deficient, making the animal even leaner and slower, and nucleic acid synthesis decreases.

Both these two kinds of drug exert a regulatory action that can help restore physiological equilibrium. This coincides with the theory of "regulating the relationship between yin and yang to reach an equilibrium." Such regulation is related to the metabolism, stocking of energy, and regulation of nerve and body fluids.

A finding is that the drug supporting yang should not be taken in summer, but in winter, because the death rate for those who take this drug in summer is higher. As for the yin-nourishing drug, it must be taken in summer, for taking it in winter may cause diarrhea and weight loss.

These findings coincide with Chinese medical theories, though the theory of yin and yang and that of deficiency and excess in Chinese medicine are more rich. The animal and man are quite different in bodily function, but the theory of yin and yang can be verified through objective things.

A work by Chen Jiewen and others of the Guangzhou College of Chinese Medicine in 1981 says that the average electric potential of the skin of patients inflicted with the deficiency syndrome of the spleen is lower than when they are quiet and stimulated by chills. The reaction of finger volume and pulse wave of patients to the stimulation is also lower than that of normal people. After convalescence and treatment, recovery is noticeable in both cases.

The skin potential of patients inflicted with a combination of the deficiency syndrome of the spleen and melancholic liver is very active, presenting multiphase waves. When they are quiet, it is higher than that of patients suffering from the deficiency syndrome of the spleen and of normal people. When suffering from chills, most maintain an active status before stimulation, and the maximum potential is almost the same as that of normal people, but higher than in patients with the deficiency syndrome of the spleen. After convalescence, the skin potential also returns to a certain extent.

Generally speaking, patients with the deficiency syndrome of the spleen usually suffer from the deficiency syndrome of yang. With a small appetite, little taste and bad digestion, they have a yellow face, are short of breath, and feel sluggish. Patients with the stagnation of the liver mostly suffer from a disorder of hepatic energy (yang in the liver). In addition to those deficiency syndromes of the spleen, there are some other indications such as uncomfortable costal ribs, swelling pain in the epigastrium, irritability, restlessness and insomnia.

A decrease in the activities of skin potential and a slow reaction to the contraction of pulsation waves of finger volume indicate in most cases a decreased function of the sympathetic nerve center and a rather strong irritability of the parasympathetic nerves. (The contraction of peripheral blood vessels, also due to the excitation of the sympathetic nerve center, is caused by the contraction of blood vessels by sympathetic nerves.) When the skin potential is very active, the excitation of the sympathetic nerve center is correspondingly high, which mobilizes the body to enhance its ability to deal with the environment and is analogized as yang. Moderate excitation of parasympathetic nerves mobilizes the internal organs to facilitate the absorption and storage of energy and is analogized as yin. These experiments suggest that patients with the deficiency of the spleen have imperiled sympathetic nerve function (the deficiency of yang), and patients with the deficiency of the spleen and the stagnation of the liver have a loss of harmony between their sympathetic and parasympathetic nerves (disharmony between yin and yang). They also show, to a certain extent, yin and yang in the *zang-fu* organs through changes in skin potential and pulsation wave in finger volume.

N. D. Cook, an American researcher, said in an article that yin and yang substances exist in the cells. These substances are mainly DNA, which belongs to yin and is concentrated in the cell's nucleus to carry hereditary information; RNA, which belongs to yang, is inside the cytoplasm to synthesize the various kinds of protein. The author added that the DNA and the RNA inside the cells enjoy an equilibrium and are stable under normal conditions, helping to maintain the synthesis of protein and the cleavage of cells. When they lose their relative equilibrium, an illness, characterized by either yin or yang, occurs, leading to disturbances in the protein synthesis and cell cleavage. Viral invasion will disturb the RNA and cause it to dissociate and perform the function of reverse transcription, causing DNA to dissociate in turn. Thus, a disturbance in protein synthesis will ensue. Tumors are also believed to have something to do with viral invasion, and are the consequence of yang predominating over yin.

Scholars studying the subject of cAMP in the cells believe that a hormone activates the adenyl cyclase on the cell membrane. This adenyl cyclase prompts adenosine triphosphatase (ATP) to drop off two phosphates to produce cAMP, and cAMP then activates protein kinase which phosphorylates protein, induces biochemical reactions, regulates cell metabolism and produces physiological functions.

Since the early 1950s, the study of cAMP has made remarkable progress, and has become an important topic in physiology, biochemistry, clinical practice, diagnosis, and therapy in molecular medicine. Goldberg, who has been mentioned earlier in this book for his creation of the "hypothesis of yin and yang," put forward an idea in 1973 after he spent much time studying cAMP and cGMP, saying that various receptors on the cell membrane, acted upon by chemical signals (the first messenger) from the outside, regulate cAMP and cGMP in the cells. They themselves act as the second messenger, again inducing the catalytic reaction in the various enzymatic cellular systems, and thereby show a different status in the functions of the cells. Based on this reasoning, Goldberg postulated his famous "hypothesis of yin and yang." CAMP prompts the decomposition of fat and glycogen, the contraction of cardiac muscle and the reduction of lysosome enzyme and histamine, and in this is similar to yang. On the other hand, cGMP prompts the synthesis of fat and glycogen, the relaxation of the cardiac muscles, and the increase of lysosome enzyme and histamine, functioning in a way similar to yin.

In an article about the deficiency syndromes in traditional Chinese medicine, Chinese researcher Xia Zongqin and his colleagues made a comparison between the content changes in cAMP in the blood plasma of patients with the deficiency of yin and those with the deficiency of yang, as well as the physiological function of cAMP and cGMP and the clinical symptoms of the deficiency of yin and yang.

A concise table published in the 11th issue, 1979, of the *Chinese Medicine Magazine* is as follow table:

With reference to cyclonucleatide, there are two kinds of receptor on the membranes of most cells: one comprises adrenergic B receptor, pancreatic hyperglycemia receptor and prostate gland E1 receptor. Once activated, this kind of receptors may enhance the cAMP level inside the cells by means of adenyl cyclase. At this time, the cGMP level inside the cells often decreases correspondingly, and the function of the cells manifests a

Organ or tissue	Physiological function of cAMP and cGMP	Clinical symptoms of the deficiency of yang (cGMP predominating)	Clinical the deficiency of symptoms of insubstantial yin (cAMP predominating)
Cardiac blood vessel	cAMP induces excitation, cGMP does not	Slender and moderate pulse	Slender and speedy pulse
Smooth muscle of alimentary canal	Excited when cAMP ascends, cGMP works on the contrary	Sticky loose stool and early morning diarrhea	Dry, constipated stool
Smooth muscle of bronchus	Excited when cAMP ascends, cGMP works on the contrary	Chronic bronchities, in severe case mostly insubstantial Yang	
Blood vessel of dermal mucous membrane	cGMP causes it to contract	Cold extremities, pale tongue, pallid face	Hot palms of hands and feet, red face and ears, red tongue
Salivary gland	CGMP promotes secretion		Parched mouth and likes drinking
Hepatic glycogen	cAMP promotes decomposition	Intolerances of cold and low basal metabolism	Afraid of heat and low sugar tolerance

state that is predominately yang.

The other kind comprises adrenergic a receptor, M-cholinergic receptor and insulin receptor. Once activated, these may enhance the level of cellular cGMP, prompting a corresponding decrease in the level of cAMP. Here the cells manifest a state similar to that of a predominance of yin. Inside the cells of a normal human body, a series of factors regulates the level of cAMP and cGMP in order to maintain a normal ratio. Scholars, proposing a "double-way control system," believe that this is similar to the theory of yin and yang; this maintains that by the mutual opposition, harmony and conditioning of yin and yang, and an organism will attain a relative equilibrium to maintain a healthy state.

Researchers chose two groups of patients. One suffered from thyroidism, which Chinese medicine attributes to the deficiency of yin. The other group had hypothyroidism, identified as the deficiency of yang. They found that if the plasma cAMP of the first group increases and cGMP decreases, the ratio of cAMP/cGMP rises; while if the plasma cAMP decreases and cGMP increases, the ratio of cAMP/cGMP decreases. That is in accord with what is said in *Huang Di Nei Jing*: "When yin is preponderant, yang will get ill, but when yang is exuberant, yin will become diseased." A wiser and deeper study of both Chinese and Western medicine will present more problems, which in turn advances the development of medicine. Molecular medicine is a highly sophisticated field that provides a modern scientific demonstration of material basis for yin and yang within an organism. It also explains the holistic concept of traditional Chinese medicine, and testifies to the concept of order and the dialectic notion of the integration of yin and yang.

The Yin-Yang Theory in Chinese Medicine

There are many connections between yin and yang in nature and those in the human body, those in the *zang-fu* organs, and those in physiology and pathology. They actively crisscross and are mutually affective and responsive. When they are harmonious and orderly, the body remains healthy; if inharmonious, the body's stability will be destroyed and diseases will then occur. The Chinese theory of treatment lies in determining the location of yin and yang before regulating their relationship for balance. This theory has long proved correct and effective, and is used as the guiding principle of traditional Chinese medicine and its methodology. However, there are people who pay little attention to those basic theories, which they say are scientifically groundless. What they are interested in are the application and research of Chinese prescriptions and herbal drugs. Of course, their application, research, summation and promotion are entirely necessary, since they contribute to the study and scientific demonstration of traditional Chinese medicine and the integration of Chinese and Western medicine in order to create a new medical science. It should be pointed out, however, that Chinese prescriptions and herbal drugs cannot be separated from their theoretical basis. For a long time, medical theory, therapeutic methods, prescriptions and herbal drugs have been part of the entire academic system. If the theory and method are neglected, prescriptions and herbal drugs cannot be accurately recognized and applied. As a result, medicine is usually prescribed and taken when just learning about the name of the disease, or Chinese medicine is taken in the same way as the Western one.

Take *Herba Ephedrae* for example. Its chemical components, molecular structure and bio-chemical actions are now quite clear. As ephedrine can excite sympathetic nerves and inhibit parasympathetic nerves, we usually use this drug to reduce fever, relax smooth muscle spasms and subdue asthma.

This research has played an important role in extending our knowledge and use of ephedra. However, if we render treatment in the light of an overall analysis of symptoms and signs, the uses of ephedra will be far more extensive than those mentioned above. In the case of a cold with excess in the exterior, hidrosis and a tense pulse, ephedra (usually matched with a cassia twig) normalizes the flow of yang-*qi* and dispels pathogenic factors from the exterior of the body, thus initiating diaphoresis, reducing fever and subduing asthma. If the deficient yang is affected by exogenous pathogenic factors, with fever and a deep pulse, the diagnosis will indicate superficial invasion. In this case, ephedra should be combined with *Radix Aconiti* and *Herba Asari* to warm yang, thus rescuing the interior and driving out the pathogenic factors. There is some difference in dosage when yang is activated and warmed. Asthma and cough are caused by unventilated energy in the lung, affected by fever and obstructed by pathogenic factors. Therefore, in order to make asthma subside and stop a cough, *Herba Ephedrae* should be combined with *Gypsum Fibrosum*. If the lung is excessive and there are symptoms of coughing and gasping for breath, it should be used with *Semen Armeniacae Amarum* to check the perverted flow of *qi*. Since one illness is cold and the other hot, the application of *Herba Ephedrae* should also be different.

Taking real symptoms and signs into account, you can find different uses for this single herb *Herba Ephedrae* and good results are gained. The dissociation of the components and structure of a herb will not offer you with knowledge about pharmaco-dynamics and indications of Chinese drugs; it is also necessary to make an analysis of the effects of different drugs under different conditions guided by the theory.

Chapter III

THE *ZANGXIANG* THEORY

Genesis

The *zangxiang* theory, otherwise known as the theory of *zang-fu* organs, is a study of the physiological functions and pathological changes of the *zang-fu* organs, *jingluo*, *jing*, *qi*, blood and body fluid, and the mutual relationship between them.

The theory derives from ancient Chinese dissection of the body. *Huang Di Nei Jing* says: "A man is covered externally with skin and flesh that can be measured and weighed. The body may be dissected to discover the strength and fragility of the *zang* organs, the size of the *fu* organs, the length of blood vessels, the clarity of blood and the density of *qi*.... All of them have an approximate number, size and length." *Huang Di Nei Jing* gives a detailed description of the *zang-fu* organs, the shape of the body, the material of the bone, and *jingluo*. As *Huang Di Nei Jing* puts it, the length from the fauces to the stomach is 1.6 feet,... the stomach winds itself but will be 2.6 feet when it is straightened,... the length of the intestine-stomach from its entrance to its outlet extends to 64.4 feet." This explains that the ratio of the length between the esophagus and the large and small intestines is 1 to 35, very close to the ratio of 1 to 37 as shown in modern anatomy. It is said in *Han Shu* ("The Book of the Han Dynasty") that the imperial physician Shang Fang dissected the corpse of Wang Sunqing and measured his five *zang* organs and blood vessels with a bamboo stick. He then said that he could have cured the diseases. This testifies to such a fact that anatomy and medicine have already been closely related for a long time. *Hou Han Shu* ("The Book of the Eastern Han Dynasty") makes some mention of the operation given by Hua Tuo (?-203), a famous surgeon in the Han Dynasty. It says:

> If a man suffers from a disease somewhere in the body that cannot be treated by means of acupuncture and medication, he should be given an operation. The method is to use the oral anesthetic *mafeisan* with rice wine, and when he gets drunk and loses consciousness, his abdomen or back is opened and something that causes trouble are taken off; if the disease is found in a place between the intestines and the stomach, he should be opened to have the sickening dregs washed away and then stitched together and smeared with sacred pastes. The cuts will heal in four or five days and the patient will recover within a month.

What Hua Tuo did 1,700 years ago is miraculous; an abdominal operation could not have been done at that time without a careful study of anatomy.

However, down to the dynasties of Wei and Jin (220-419), the feudal ethical code became all the more cruel. Such filial creeds as that body, hairs and skin given by parents should not be destroyed and impaired, and many others, seriously arrested the development of anatomical science. The following story is recorded in *Song Shu* ("The Book of the Song Dynasty"). A man named Tang Ci living during the Southern Dynasties (420-589) fell ill after drinking too much wine, and vomited two dozen worms. Before dying, he told his wife to have his corpse dissected. She did what her husband asked to do, and her son made no objection to it. That was said "to have hurt Tang's five *zang* organs," and both Tang's wife and son, accused of being "unfilial to his father," were put to death. This kind of feudal code of ethics produced a harmful influence over the development of human anatomy and the spread of anesthesia in surgery. Achievements in this field were not transmitted to later generations and almost fell into oblivion.

It should be pointed out that the *zangxiang* theory does not principally focus on the description or elucidation of the shape and state of the *zang-fu* organs and their anatomical positions. In terms of modern anatomical morphology, these descriptions are not only rather immature, but are even wrong in certain cases. What is most important is its knowledge of the mutual relationship and conditioning of the physiology and pathology of the *zang-fu* organs under the guidance of the theories of yin and yang and *wuxing*. Chinese medicine, in both theory and in practice, pays great attention to *qi*, which is believed to be the key to life. As an old saying goes, *qi* imparts a physique to the human being. When *qi* assembles, the physique will exist; when it disperses, the physique will perish. Lay people are accustomed to take the cessation of *qi* (meaning breath here, the carrier of *qi*) as the sign of death. We know that human metabolism, which reflects the activity of life, is a process of assimilation and dissimilation. Assimilation means absorbing nutritious substances from the surroundings and also a certain quantity of *qi*. Dissimilation is the process by which an organism decomposes its own substance, releasing *qi* needed for the activities of life, while reducing the decomposed materials. Both are no other than oxidation and deoxidation of the various nutritious substances. An organism continuously carries on the commutation of oxygen and carbon dioxide; when this process stops, metabolism stops and life ceases. Chinese medicine uses the term "qi" to express this special feature of life and the function of *qi* to express the active mechanism of the body.

Chinese medicine has studied *qi* and the function of *qi* in physiology and pathology, and has succeeded in finding effective methods of recognizing them in order to treat the diseases of the function of *qi*. This theory is a rare treasure. Since the founding of the People's Republic of China in 1949, great efforts have been made to study the *jingluo* system in China, especially in terms of anatomical histology. However, no anatomical histological things along *jingluo* and acupuncture points have been found. Therefore, some people do not accept the existence of *jingluo* or the reliability of the *jingluo* theory. However, extensive clinical practice has proven again and again that the *jingluo* theory is an objective truth. How can we find a solution to these mutually contradictory facts? As a matter of fact, what is treated by this theory is mainly the *qi* in *jingluo*. Now *qi* can of course exist only in the living body; to search for active *qi* in a corpse would be like "climbing up a tree to catch fish," as the Chinese proverb says. We also know that theory and method are closely related, and that different theoretical systems need different research methods. In studying the theoretical system of Chinese medicine that is quite different from Western medicine, we must devise methods that will fit with it better. This will promote research and succeed in making a breakthrough in the work. For instance, the recent use of electrophysiology and biochemical tests to study Chinese medicine has been proven very effective.

When traditional Chinese medicine had no knowledge of modern anatomy, histology, physiology or pathology, how could people have learned about the physiological functions and pathological changes of the *zang-fu* organs, as well as the relationship between them only by means of the *zangxiang* theory? It is recorded in *Su Wen* ("Plain Questions"), a chapter in *Huang Di Nei Jing*, that the Emperor asked "What about *zangxiang*?" Wang Bing, a famous physician and annotator of *Huang Di Nei Jing* in the Tang Dynasty (618-907), annotated this sentence by saying: "*Xiang* (manifestation) can be read outside." Zhang Jingyue said more clearly: "The *zang* organs exist inside but express their images outside, so we have the name *zangxiang.*" Exploring and recognizing the variegated phenomena to be reflected outside the body through repeated practice, observation and thinking, people have become clear about the *zangxiang* theory. Recently, scientists have applied cybernetics to explain traditional Chinese medicine regarding the *zang-fu* organs, on the assumption that they cannot be seen superficially. It is like an unopened black box. We put certain information already known to us into the box. This acts upon certain aspects inside the box and delivers information to us from within it. The inner secrets can be gradually explored and made known from the information obtained after applying related knowledge already available and comparing and analyzing their various relations. *Huang Di Nei Jing* has this to say about this method: "The sun and the moon, the water and the mirror, the drum and the sound are all good illustrations. The brightness of the sun and the moon does not deviate from the shadow, the observation of water and the mirror does not deviate from the physique, and the knock of the drum is immediately followed by the sound. When you shout, an echo will return. In all these cases, the reaction is complete.... The abundant brightness cannot be shadowed, because yin (shadow) and yang (light) will never perish. We should observe the patient from all aspects, feel the pulse to verify the symptoms and master the situation with our eyes, as clean water and a bright mirror never distort the shape of the physique. If *wusheng* is not articulate, *wuse* is not clear and the five *zang* organs are vibrating, then there are mutual interferences between the outside and inside, just as the drum will inevitably respond to the knock of the stick, the sound will have its echo and the shadow should conform to the physique. Therefore, when the object is far away, then observe the exterior to conjecture what is inside; when the object is near by, then observe the interior to conjecture what is outside. This is the so-called response of yin and yang and the boundaries of heaven and earth." This vividly describes how the structure and function of the *zang* organs inside the human body can be reflected in the information of *wuse, wusheng*, etc., that are expressed externally. The structure and function can be vividly laid bare if all the information is examined and summarized in accordance with the fundamental law of the integration of yin and yang. This is the method adopted by Chinese medicine in order to deduce what is inside from outside, by examining the symptom-complex to find out the cause. This is a special feature of the *zangxiang* theory, and is similar to the information method of the black box theory. For instance, people have realized through long-term practice that when they become chilled, their fine hairs stand on end; they are then liable to catch a cold and cough. If sudorific and the drug to ventilate the lung are administered, the disease can be cured. From this relationship of cause and effect, people have gradually realized that "the lungs, skin, and hair maintain a relationship of exterior and interior" and that "a cough comes from vibrations in the lungs."

When my grandson was one year old he was very healthy and lively. Once, after I had not seen him for three months, I found his skin and hair dry. He coughed and panted and was in a sluggish mood. Upon inquiring, I was told he had caught a cold two months earlier and had developed a fever and cough. After he was given penicillin, the fever was allayed but the cough and stridor persisted for a long time, and his fingers were purple. This was due to the stasis of wind and cold in his lungs which had not been ventilated and dissolved; the protracted stasis had induced the fever. After I administered a decoction consisting of *Herba Ephedrae, Semen Armeniacae Amarae, Gypsum Fibrosum* and *Radix Glycyrrhizae*, the cough and the stridor disappeared. One week later, his skin and hair were sleek and glossy again, and he was as lively as before. It is through such practice that people have accumulated the medical knowledge which gradually formed the *zangxiang*.

Marxist theory believes that human knowledge comes

from social practice. During the process of practice, people sense the phenomena of objective things of the external world, including their own selves. They acquire empirical knowledge in the form of sense perception, consciousness, and ideas. When knowledge passes through comparison and discrimination, analysis and synthesis, and abstraction and generalization, it gradually becomes refined and more accurate. Accurate thinking built on accurate perception will correctly reflect the essence of objective things and will conform to objective regularities. If perception and thinking don't completely reflect reality, the knowledge acquired will be one-sided.

In ancient China, scientific and technological thought were still inchoate, and there was both accurate and inaccurate knowledge of human body. For this reason, it is necessary to sort out and systematize traditional Chinese medicine, selecting its valuable parts and discarding the rest. While we disapprove of the negation of the theory of visceral manifestations of traditional medicine, we also disapprove of conservative thinking which cherishes broken and worn-out things and does not try positively to systematize, study and elevate Chinese medicine. Traditional Chinese medicine has been developed under the guidance of naive dialectics through the social practice of millions of people over the centuries. It is generally recognized that the roads to truth have been constantly opened up in the course of practice. Even if certain theories have proven effective in medical practice, we should study them seriously, attempt to explore their mystery, and finally preserve their essence.

The development of science has made man's field of vision wider than ever. What seemed inconceivable in the past is understandable and clear now. So many things that are not quite clear to us now will prove their worth in scientific development as long as they can stand the test of actual practice. The objective world is infinite and human ability to understand the world is also infinite. The part of the world we know today is certainly far smaller than the unknown part. Therefore, we must not deny the existence of those things which science still cannot interpret and thereby repudiate them as unscientific or denounce them as absurd. The attitude of repudiation and denunciation is principally due to the lack of an accurate understanding of the relationship between relative truth and absolute truth. If this narrow attitude is not criticized, it will block the chain of thinking and obstruct the progress of science.

Modern scientists are using 1,000-year-old trees to study the activities of sunspots; the annual rings show the growth of the tree, which is directly related to the sun's activities. Within these rings, scientists have discovered radiocarbon produced by cosmic rays, with most coming from the sun. With this information scientists can estimate the changes in the sun's activities.

Is there a relationship between the internal organs and the body surface that would explain the *zangxiang* even more clearly? This question is now being actively explored in China. According to *The Journal of Traditional Chinese Medicine*, internal organs, if diseased or damaged, may lead to an abnormality or tenderness in the corresponding acupoints. The formation of a low electric resistance point on the auricle can be verified by means of an embedded electrode as shown in an experiment at the Department of Biology of Shanghai Normal University some years ago. This point is mainly due to the centripetal attack of wandering nerves caused by pathological stimulation, while the sympathetic nerves are the principal channels that transmit the pathological information. Researchers at the Beijing Medical College also discovered after studying the basic principles of acupuncture anesthesia that if the sympathetic nerves are retained, the relationship between the stomach and the skin of the auricle remains normal; but if they are severed, this relationship is attenuated. From this, it can be seen that the fiber of the sympathetic nerve is one of the material bases of the relationship between internal organs and the body surface. Of ourse, such experimental research is only a beginning; the issue itself is far more complicated. It shows, however, that research on the *zangxiang* theory has already had broad prospects opened before it.

It should also be pointed out that since traditional Chinese methods of observing and studying the physiology and pathology of the internal organs are quite different from those adopted by Western medicine, differences will naturally exist in their understanding of the same object; accordingly, different theories will form. Scholars integrated Chinese and Western medicine in the late Qing Dynasty (1644-1911) and adopted methods that were not correct. They usually made use of theories of Chinese or Western medicine to interpret Western or Chinese theories, and in so doing, they unavoidably often adopted things uncritically, spending great efforts and accomplishing very little. This practice still exists today, along with the problem. The integration of Chinese and Western medicine will demand much more study and research, involving methods of thought and theoretical systems; simple comparisons will not contribute much. Moreover, some maintain that Western medicine has passed examination by modern science, while many traditional Chinese theories are incompatible with Western knowledge. They therefore doubt the scientific nature of Chinese medicine. Marxism, however, believes that practice is the sole criterion to test the truth. Since therapeutic practice under the guidance of the *zangxiang* theory has already shown its excellent effects, we should first discard the suspicious or contemptuous attitude towards it and then devote painstaking labor to integrate Chinese and Western medicine.

Tentative Comment on "Reverberating View of Inside Scene"

How did Chinese medicine develop such a peculiar method of recognizing the *zang-fu* organs and *jingluo* in the human body? What did the Chinese people use to recognize the body and its environment, the *zang-fu* organs, *jingluo*, *qi*, blood, body fluid and *jing*, and the configurative force and physique, as well as their functions and holistic relationship? Many of these things, although not yet proven by modern scientific and technological means, have displayed convincing results in clinical practice. For instance, the *jingluo* theory and the treatment of diseases by acupuncture and moxibustion have been widely known and popularly received. However, up to now and despite much research, the substance and mechanism of *jingluo* and acupoints have not yet been clarified.

Practice is the source of knowledge. Learning is always a developing process of practice, learning, repeated practice, and repeated learning. Learning starts from practice in production, in living, in health protection and in the prevention and treatment of diseases. Chinese traditional medicine has accumulated knowledge and has even made use of the method of the black box theory to gradually form its own theory. Since it has its own original theories and specific knowledge, however, does it also possess its own original method of learning? This section of the book will explore whether a method of learning— the so-called "reverberating view of the inside scene" or "introscanning"— actually exists.

The term "reverberating view of the inside scene" originated in *Qi Jing Ba Mai Kao* ("A Study on the Eight Extra Channels") written by Li Shizhen, a well-known pharmacologist in the Ming Dynasty (1368-1644). Li said: "The tunnel to the inside scene can only be observed through the reverberator." Only those who have acquired certain training and mental cultivation (such as *qigong* masters and meditators) can see introspectively ("reverberatively"), observe and recognize the inside scene of the *zang-fu* organs and the tunnels of *jingluo*. There have been repeated accounts in Chinese history books of instances of the "reverberating view of the inside scene" or "introscanning." *Shi Ji* ("The Records of the Historian"), for example, has something to say about Bian Que, a famous physician in the Period of Warring States (475-221 B.C.). Once he went to make diagnosis of Qi Huan Hou. When meeting with the duke, Bian Que told him that a disease had already existed in him, and that would spread from skin into blood vessels, intestines, stomach and finally the vitals. The duke refused to accept treatment, for he did not believe what the physician had told him. Nevertheless, the diagnosis was correct, and the duke died before long. There have been plenty of records in various dynasties about *qigong* practitioners aware of the circulation of inner *qi* in the body, able to make it circulate along the *Ren* and *Du* channels to form a small *zhoutian* (circulation of *qi*) and along the twelve regular channels and the eight extra channels" to form a large *zhoutian*. They are even said to be capable of directing *qi* to the site of an illness in order to cure it. This treating method has been passed down from ancient times and is still widely used today. It has attracted great interest and instituted research all over the world.

As a matter of fact, our knowledge of *jingluo* came from daily practice. Certain seats of foci were found to be able of curing some diseases and radiating *qi* towards certain positions or routes inside the body; it was on this basis that experiences were accumulated and developed. In time, the related seats were connected, and knowledge of *jingluo* was then obtained. Among the medical literature unearthed from the Han tombs at Mawangdui near Changsha, capital of Hunan Province in 1972, however, *Zu Bi Shi Yi Mai Jiu Jing* ("Moxibustion Classic of Eleven Pulses on Arms and Feet") and *Yin Yang Shi Yi Mai Jiu Jing* ("Moxibustion Classic of Eleven Yin and Yang Pulses"), which were believed to appear earlier than *Huang Di Nei Jing*, only described the circulation of *jingluo*, not the "induction" seats of foci. This shows that the knowledge of seats of foci was not acquired during the prevention and treatment of diseases prior to the discovery of *jingluo* from the relationship between these seats. What, then, is the source of this knowledge? This reminded us of what Li Shizhen said: "The tunnel to the inside scene can only be observed through the reverberator."

Since 1949, there have been repeated reports about the people sensitive to *jingluo*, who feel the flow of *qi* in the channels. Even though most know nothing about medicine or the seats of foci of *jingluo*, the flowing routes they described were the same as those explained in the *jingluo* theory. *Qi* can also be detected with a special apparatus. When you detect the bodily position where *qi* has arrived by means of the infrared thermal imaging system, you can find that it has a higher temperature than other places.

The method of learning about the "reverberating view of the inside scene" or "introscanning," mentioned in traditional literature, is one aspect of perceptual knowledge. It comes from perception of the internal phenomena of the human body under specific conditions through specific information. Such perceptual knowledge will gradually become rational and thus one phase of the *zangxiang* theory. This channel to knowledge cannot be denied without making an analysis and investigation, because failure to do so will block the way which might lead to a new realm of knowledge.

The "reverberating view of the inside scene" realized through *qigong* deals with a complicated movement in the natural world— a reciprocal movement between consciousness and the human body. Since both the body and consciousness are the products of evolutionary development, we are probably now on the verge of a breakthrough in natural science and medicine. Attention should be given to the following points if we are to speed up this breakthrough.

First, we should stand on the foundation of the present scientific theories and technology yet constantly try to expand the field of basic medical theories. For instance, how can we recognize on the basis of holistic connections the interaction between the body and the mind? Here in traditional Chinese medicine and *qigong*, spirit and matter, and consciousness and flesh are regarded as an interacting totality. This has been the starting point of the study and will present a new prospect for an advanced understanding of the movement of human life. A *qigong* master, for example, places a 1,000-1,500-kg slab of stone on his stomach and then has it knocked with a large, heavy hammer, but the master remains unscathed when the slabstone is broken into pieces. How can he sustain such heavy pressure? This is because of an amazing relationship between the body and the mind and between flesh and consciousness developed in *qigong*, in which the aim is to direct *qi* in the body and create a functional mood. Isn't this worthy of our exploration and investigation? The more we discover all the *qi* functions in the body which cannot be explained by existing scientific theories, the more we should grope for their scientific regularities. We should not lightly repudiate their objective existence simply because they are beyond the bounds of explanation by existing scientific theories.

Second, since theory and method are closely interrelated, different systems of science and learning have different methods of research and experiment. The science of the human body should not be content with existing medical research. For instance, the use of animal models will not fulfill the requirements of research in new areas. We must instead creatively design new research projects and experimental methods.

Research requires joint cooperation of many disciplines and joint participation of concerned scientists from different fields. In his thesis *Expand the Basic Research in the Science of the Human Body*, Prof. Qian Xuesen proposes a series of thought-provoking ideas. He maintains that the human body is a highly complicated large-scale system in which, in addition to functional moods like waking, sleeping and hypnosis, there is the functional mood of *qigong*. He maintains that the basic study of the human body should concentrate on its various functional moods and the influence of consciousness on the body on the one hand, and the circulation of *qi* in the body should not be thought of as a matter running along the channels but a perception expressed by the human body through consciousness on the other. The external *qi* discharged by a *qigong* master acts upon living and nonliving things. That is a kind of resonance produced after the large-scale system of the body is expanded. The connections between any part of this system are indissoluble; it coincides with the basic study of quantum mechanics and the viewpoint of integration of nature and mankind. Professor Qian points out that it is compatible with the development of modern science in studying the body. He believes that the trio— the working of *qigong*, Chinese medical theory and the body's idiosyncratic function— fosters the fundamental principle in the science of the human body. In his thesis, Professor Qian elucidates the necessity of multiple disciplines collaborating to study this problem.

Consequently, the "reverberating view of the inside scene" is an important issue, which we expect will return to the forefront of science. Latent functions, hidden deep inside the human body, will contribute to further understanding of the riddle of the "black box."

The *Zangxiang* Theory from the Viewpoint of Yin and Yang

The *zangxiang* theory takes the yin-yang theory as its guide, along with concepts of interconnection, inter-inhibition, movement and change. It therefore constitutes a holistic view of balance and order.

To begin with, the theory believes that the *zang* organs belong to yin and the *fu* organs to yang. There is a paragraph in *Huang Di Nei Jing* which deals with the basic functions of the *zang-fu* organs in broad line, saying: "The so-called five *zang* organs collect *jing* but do not reduce it, and thus are full but not substantial. The six *fu* organs transform and dissolve but do not store, and thus are substantial but not full." This generalization still holds considerable guiding significance in clinical practice. Take for example the treatment of an acute problem in the abdomen, like appendicitis and intestinal obstruction. Purgation was usually banned to promote intestinal peristalsis in Western medicine, for that this would run the risk of stimulating perforation and diffusion in the inflamed section of the intestines. Great successes have been made in this field by combining Chinese and Western medicine since 1949, and it is by means of purgation that many people have been cured of acute abdomen. This is because traditional Chinese medicine maintains that stomach, large and small intestines and gallbladder are all among the *fu* organs whose function is to reduce and clear, transform and dissolve things, instead of storing them. Acute inflammation and obstruction in the intestines will therefore disrupt their ability to transform, dissolve and clear, and a morbid state will naturally result. If normal functions are to be restored, attention must be riveted on "purgation." For the past 2,000 years, traditional Chinese medicine has used purgation to treat similar syndromes in the *fu* organs. This is mentioned in *Shang Han Lun* in which two kinds of decoction are prescribed, and they are still used today, with minor changes in dosage, to treat certain acute abdomen syndromes.

One day in the winter of 1965, a 20-year-old lad in Hunan suffered from acute appendicitis. The pain was intense and lasted throughout the night. He was rushed to the hospital, where he was told that he must have an operation at once. Unwilling to do so, he and his family came to me for consultation. At first, I advised them to have the operation, but they refused again, insisting on having a try at Chinese medicine. I have no other choice but to make diagnosis of him. His pulse was found to be tight, swift, tense and speedy, and the coating on his tongue yellow and thick. He bent from the waist and knees because his abdomen was distended and ached terribly. I then prescribed four doses of herbal drug consisting of *Radix et Rhizoma Rhei, Cortex Moutan Radicis, Semen Persicae, Semen Benincasae, Natrii Sulfas, Herba Oldenlandiae, Fructus Aurantii Immaturus* and *Cortex Magnoliae Officinalis*. After one dose, his abdominal distention and pain subsided, and was entirely cured after four doses. No recurrence has taken place since. The effect, therefore, was realized by administering a decoction whose function is to reduce and purge. This further testifies to the inexhaustible genius of Chinese traditional medicine.

Based on the unity of yin and yang, the *zangxiang* theory tells not only about a general cognition that the *zang* organs belong to yin and the *fu* ones to yang, but also more, showing that every *zang* or *fu* organ has its own yin and yang. When yin and yang of the various *zang-fu* organs are in a state of unity and relative equilibrium, the *zang-fu* organs themselves are healthy. If the *zang* or *fu* organs are impaired, or if yin and yang between them is unbalanced, a pathological condition in that particular organ will occur. For instance, if yin of the heart is deficient, the patient will most likely have symptoms of palpitation, irritability, amnesia, insomnia and dreaminess; if yang of the heart is deficient, then nervousness, short breath, cold limbs, cold body, slender and weak pulse or slow pulse with an irregular beat may ensue. The general therapeutic principle of Chinese medicine for treating visceral diseases, therefore, remains that of readjusting the *zang-fu* organs, as well as yin and yang, so as to replenish what is lacking and eliminate what is excessive in order to achieve balance.

The *zangxiang* theory systematically and dialectically considers the mutual connection and inhibition between things.

1) The interrelation and inter-inhibition between the *zang* and *fu* organs. Consider the statement that "the heart is warmth in heaven, fire on earth, and summer in terms of the season, maize of the cereal and vegetable of the shallot." This explains that the heart is as lively as fire and is the source of motive power for the whole body. The weather in summer is good for those with heart diseases, but the chilly winter is disadvantageous. Excessive heat, a high fever, or excessive sweating due to deficient yang, however, will cause discomfort. (Sweat is the fluid of the heart.) Maize and shallots have a close connection with the heart, and ancient Chinese advocated "eating more shallots in case of heart disease." Nowadays, it is clinically proved that the shallot is one of effective drugs for heart disease. This testifies to the fact that there is a close relationship between the heart and the outside world.

In the prevention and treatment of diseases, Chinese medicine pays close attention to the relationship between the *zang-fu* organs and the natural world. For instance, spring is windy, and as it is apt to agitate the endogenous hepatic wind. Chinese physicians maintain that patients suffering from mental or nervous diseases, which are related to this wind, should guard against their attack. On sweltering summer days when *qi* is easily impaired and the heat stroke incurred, pay attention to the prevention of acute febrile diseases; if the summer is quite long, and the spleen and stomach are impaired by heat and dampness, take some preventive measures against infectious diseases in the digestive system between summer and autumn. Autumnal dryness is liable to hurt the lungs, and so cough and asthma should be prevented, and tuberculous patients must be careful about their illness. Winter is an attribute of water, so attention should be given to the prevention of asthma when the kidney fails to absorb enough *qi* due to a lack of renal water.

2) The interrelations between the *zang* organs and their manifestations. The conditions of *zang* and *fu* organs are often reflected in some part of the body or on its sur-

face. For instance, the orifice of the heart is the tongue, its taste is bitter, its fluid is sweat and its health is reflected in the face. The tongue is related to the heart. Thus, if the cardiac fire is too vigorous, the tip of the tongue will be a dark red. If yang of the heart is deficient, the tongue will be fat, large and whitish. If the blood in the heart is silted up, the tongue will be dark. The faces of people with heart disease usually look very bad, and people with deficient yang of the heart usually sweat spontaneously; during heart failure, in fact profuse sweating often occurs. Those with heart disease often feel a pain at a place that the heart and pericardium channels run or the *xinshu* acupoint in the back. The general condition of the heart can be diagnosed through the abnormalities of the external parts of the body related to the heart by observation, auscultation and olfaction and interrogation.

That the kidney has its specific body opening in the ears may be cited as another instance. Clinically, nephritic patients, especially those suffering from renal failure, often complain of tinnitus and deafness. The auricles of patients with the deficiency syndrome of the kidney often look shriveled, thin and withered. Moreover, their hair falls off or becomes withered or white prematurely. The reason is that the splendor of the kidney is usually reflected at the hair. Again, "the kidney governs the bone," and "the essence of the bone is the pupil." Therefore, the pupils of patients suffering from the deficiency syndrome of the kidney are dilated, large and listless, and their vision is weak. In most cases, they adapt to the pills made up of *Fructus Lycii, Flos Chrysanthemi* and *Radix Rehmanniae*, a prescription used to tonify the kidney. As the "kidney is in charge of the bone," clinically, the bones of renal patients are often soft, decalcified, and easily fractured. Tonifying the kidney in cases of infantile chondropathy often produces striking effects.

The physical complexion does not reflect the appearance of a specific organ but also reveals the condition of the multiple connections and movements enjoyed by that particular organ with other *zang* organs, *jingluo*, *qi* and blood. The tongue, for one, is said to be the sprout of the heart, meaning that to a certain extent one can perceive the condition of the heart from texture, color and form of the tongue. Moreover, the tongue's condition (flourishing or withering), color (red, crimson, purple, blue or black), texture (tough or delicate, fat or lean, with bristle-like coating, cracked, swollen or shriveled), and phases (soft, hard, trembling, flaccid, askew, oblique, shrunken, stretching and wagging) also reflect the general condition of the whole body and the other organs.

Different parts of the tongue can be used to diagnose different *zang* organs. The center of the tongue, for instance, reflects the spleen and the stomach, the fundus reflects the kidney and the gallbladder, the two sides reflect the liver and the bile, and the tip reflects the heart and lung. The problems reflected in the changes of the tongue color and texture are very complicated. A whitish coating is caused by the invasion of wind and cold; yellow is mostly due to the stagnancy of stomach or dryness and accumulation in the large intestine; and white, glossy coating indicates that the spleen has been affected by dampness and phlegm. Obviously, these manifestations are not those of a single factor or lineal cause and effect, but are instead composite expressions of the interactions of several factors, variables and regularities. This applies also to such other expressions as the pulse, complexion, facial expression, etc. Historical conditions prevented Chinese medicine from adopting modern scientific means to diagnose the functions of internal organs; instead, it could only study the interior by closely observing the exterior, and more intently, in fact, than other medical sciences have. This valuable method should be carefully studied and developed.

For instance, though sweating is a common phenomenon, any minute difference in its occurrence (such as time, location and quality of the sweating) can reflect different physiological and pathological states. Sweating due to noxious wind often signifies the deficiency of the exterior, spontaneous sweating in the daytime is mostly due to the deficiency of yang, sweating during sleep is caused by the deficiency of yin, and profuse dripping sweat indicates the deficiency and decline of yang-*qi*. Fever with profuse sweating is due to heat in the Stomach Channel of Foot-*Yangming*, while yellow sweat may be caused by stagnant dampness. If the sweat is clean and thin like water, it is mostly due to the deficiency syndrome; sweat which smells like fish or mutton is caused by wind, dampness and heat fermenting in the skin; sticky and greasy sweet is a sign of prostration; and oily sweat is mostly a symptom of approaching death. If only the forehead sweats, it is most likely due to fainting caused by the deficiency of yang; if only the feet, it is most likely due to dampness and heat in the lower cavity. If one side of the body sweats, this is probably due to the breakdown of the balance between yin and yang.

Even though modern science uses instruments to simulate the operation of the four methods of diagnosis in Chinese medicine, they cannot replace these methods. For instance, the sphygmophone, an instrument for measuring pulse rate cannot easily reflect the interactions of the multiple factors, variables and regularities in the relationships of *zangxiang* mentioned above. Of course, computer technology will certainly help solve problems in this field; indeed, the whole set of theories, methods, diagnosis and therapeutic technology of Chinese medicine should be written into a computer program. Such sense perceptions as sight, hearing and touch could be simulated, and their synthesis and analysis could be conducted with a view to producing a computer function capable of recognizing the interaction of factors in *zangxiang*. Several problems in this area await study and investigation.

3) The relationship between the *zang* organs, between the *zang* and *fu* organs and between the *fu* organs.

Chinese medicine associates the five *zang* organs with *wuxing*. The function of *wuxing* in generating, overcoming, inhibiting and resolving reflects a relationship of interconnection and mutual inhibition and generation between the *zang* and *fu* organs. Besides, the relationship between the *zang* and *fu* organs can been seen both outside and inside. For instance, the lung is associated with the large intestine, the heart with the small intestine, the liver with the bile, the spleen with the stomach, and the kidney with the gallbladder. That is why they, along with yin and yang, are considered as a closely connected and harmonious organism.

4) The relationship between the *zang-fu* organs and mental activity. Although thought and emotion are guided by the brain, traditional Chinese medicine nevertheless maintains that the heart governs mental activity and is the principal of the various organs. According to *Huang Di Nei Jing*, the heart is the chief of the five *zang* and six *fu* organs. When one grieves, laments, worries or is in a melancholy mood, the heart will stir. When the heart stirs, the *zang* and *fu* organs will shake. In addition, traditional Chinese medicine believes that the heart stores the divine spirit: in ambition, it is happiness; in motion, melancholy. The liver stores the mental spirit: in ambition, it is anger; in motion, grasping. The kidney holds ambition: in ambition, it is fear; in motion, trembling. The lung holds bodily spirit: in ambition, it is melancholy; in motion, coughing. The spleen stocks intent: in ambition, it is thinking; in motion, retching. In this manner, traditional Chinese medicine connects various mental faculties and emotions with the functions and conditions of the different *zang* and *fu* organs.

A good psychological interpretation of the divine, mental and bodily spirits, along with intent and ambition, was made in *Huang Di Nei Jing*: "Therefore, what is inborn is called *jing*. Two kinds of *jing* fight to embrace each other to form the divine spirit. What accompanies *jing* in entering and exiting is called the bodily spirit.

Therefore, what takes charge of things is called the heart; what the heart considers is called the intent; what the intent aims at is called ambition. To meditate on the existence and possible changes is called thinking; to aspire through thinking about the distant future is called concern; to dispose of things out of concern is called intelligence." In this way the relationship between the physical body and mental activity is built on a materialistic foundation.

In the field of pathology, Chinese medicine emphatically stresses the pathological action caused by the seven emotions when they are excessive: joy, anger, anxiety, worry, grief, apprehension and fright. It maintains that such excess will not merely hurt the heart and spirit— the central nervous system— but will also directly and indirectly afflict the relevant *zang-fu* organs. For instance, immense anger hurts the liver, great joy impairs the heart, terrible fear harms the kidney, deep sorrow damages the lung, and excessive thinking injures the spleen. As *Huang Di Nei Jing* states: "I know that all diseases originate from genuine *qi*.... When one is angry, his genuine *qi* will be affronted; at the worst, he will vomit blood and have diarrhea, thus causing the ascent of genuine *qi*. When one is happy, genuine *qi* is mild and the aspiration tends to be optimistic; both constructive and defensive *qi* flows smoothly and genuine *qi* runs slowly. When one is grievous, his heart beats quickly, his lungs expand and their lobes rise, the upper cavity is blocked and both constructive and defensive *qi* cannot disperse. Accordingly, heat concentrates and genuine *qi* vanishes. When one fears, the *jing* retreats... and the upper cavity closes. If it is closed, genuine *qi* turns back, causing the lower cavity to inflate, and the flow of genuine *qi* stops.... When one is frightened, the heart is deprived of its support and the divine spirit finds nowhere to reside, while worry drifts and genuine *qi* is deranged.... When one thinks, the heart has something to rest on, and the divine spirit finds somewhere to reside, and genuine *qi* does not circulate." In treating diseases caused by aspiration and emotion, Chinese medicine emphasizes the regulation of genuine *qi*. It maintains, moreover, that psychotherapy should be used mostly to cure these diseases by changing one's viewpoint in life. If, contrary to this teaching, "addiction and sexual desires are not controlled and concerns and worries are endless, then *jing* and genuine *qi* will slacken and deteriorate, while nourishment and defense will be removed. By that time, the divine spirit will leave and the diseases will not be cured," as explained in *Huang Di Nei Jing*.

In addition to paying attention to "diseases caused by melancholia," Chinese medicine also stresses "melancholy caused by diseases," that is, nervous and psychic diseases caused by derangement of the functions of the *zang-fu* organs. Therefore, Chinese medicine embodies various methods, not only of removing melancholy to cure diseases, but also removing diseases to cure melancholy, that is, to cure the derangement of the *zang* and *fu* functions with a view to curing nervous and psychic diseases. We frequently receive patients suffering from neurosis, who ordinarily think too much about things and are distressed. They gradually become depressed and anxious, with symptoms of palpitation, insomnia, liability to be frightened, lack of appetite, mental sluggishness, short breath and weakness. Since Chinese medicine maintains that this is due to an impairment of the heart and the spleen. In addition to counseling, it uses prescriptions to cure these organs. If such recipes as a spleen rehabilitation decoction are prescribed to treat the heart and spleen, neurosis will also be cured at the same time.

5) The interconnection between the *zang* and *fu* organs on the one hand, and *jing*, genuine *qi*, blood and fluid on the other. *Jing, qi*, blood and fluid constitute the functions of the *zang-fu* organs, and additionally connect the *zang* and *fu* organs and make organs, tissues and cells an organism. Traditional Chinese medicine also believes that there are specific connections between *jing, qi*,

blood and fluid on the one hand, and the *zang* and *fu* organs on the other. For instance, there are two kinds of *jing*, one coming inborn and the other produced from food through its circulation and dissolution after it has been transported to the various *zang-fu* organs. The kidney contains both the congenital and acquired *jing*; hence the saying: "kidney stores *jing*." If the kidney did not store it, the body's constitution would deteriorate, all bodily functions would decline and the configurative force would become listless. Therefore, a cure should start with the reinforcement of the kidney.

Traditional medicine additionally believes that genuine *qi* is in the kidney, thoracic *qi* accumulates in the lungs, constructive *qi* circulates in the channels, and while the source of defensive *qi* is in the lower cavity (kidney), it is propagated in the middle cavity (spleen) and developed in the upper (lungs).

There are the specific interconnections of the heart in generating, the liver in storing and the spleen in controlling blood. Therefore, the heart, liver and spleen should be taken into account in treating blood diseases and menstrual disorders.

Traditional medicine maintains that the spleen is in charge of circulation and digestion and transportation, the lung cleanses the inspired air and keep *qi* flowing downward, and the kidney governs water metabolism. So, the treatment of dropsy usually starts with diagnosis of the lung, spleen and kidney. Thus, in cases of primary acute nephritis, fever, aversion to cold, incontinence, edema, etc., the following prescriptions are prepared: *Herba Ephedrae, Radix Forsythiae, Semen Phaseoli* and *yuebi*, all of them being decoctions. In addition, chronic nephritis should be treated in the light of the spleen and kidney.

Jing, qi, blood and body fluid are connected and always in motion— ascending, descending, reducing and absorbing. Under normal conditions, lucid yang is at the top, turbid yin is below, while the spleno-gastric *qi* is the pivot for raising the lucid and suppressing the turbid. "The *qi* of the *ying* system flows in a natural direction while that of the *wei* system runs adversely." When both kinds of *qi* are in harmony, the skin is healthy. Reduction and absorption form an organism's concrete channel of metabolism: Food is assimilated and dissimilated. Inhaling oxygen and exhaling carbon dioxide are indispensable to the respiration of cells and transmutation of *qi*. If the ascent and descent are not regulated, the lucid and the turbid interfere with each other, *qi* of the *ying* system and that of the *wei* are unbalanced, reduction and absorption are disturbed, and the organism becomes diseased. Because ascent, descent, reduction and absorption are closely connected, they surely produce an effect upon one another.

Qi is very important in traditional Chinese medicine. Many philosophers in ancient China shared the point of view that the movements of all things in the world were said to be produced or caused by genuine *qi*. They maintained that the source of the cosmos was *qi*, not spirit. In his book *Lun Heng*, Wang Chong (27-97), a philosopher in the Han Dynasty, said: "The birth of all things in the world is endowed with *qi*." In the opinion of Wang Chong, human life and mental activity took "genuine *qi*" as their material basis. He said in an article that genuine *qi* became extinct immediately upon death, and without *qi*, life would disappear. Considerable literature exists in Chinese philosophy on material monist thoughts like those of Wang Chong. In fact, the monism in traditional Chinese medicine began much earlier and was richer in content. However, researchers in the history of philosophical thought have little to say on this subject.

Huang Di Nei Jing vividly explains that the beginning and the source of all things in the cosmos is *qi*: its spread and circulation give rise to the movement and development of things in the world. The passage ends by saying: "In the atmosphere, it is *qi*; on the earth, it assumes a physical shape. The *qi* and the shape induce each other and resolve themselves to produce all things in the world."

Genuine *qi* in human body is sophisticated and subtle substance, as is its function. It is the source of the metabolism. "Mankind is given birth by the heaven and the earth and brought up by the four seasons." *Qi* is the foundation of mutual relationship between the body and its surroundings. There are two kinds of *qi* in heaven and earth: yin-*qi* and yang-*qi*. The activity of *qi*, an integration of yin and yang, is the foundation of the human body. It is on this holistic foundation that traditional medicine recognizes the specificity of the *zang* and *fu* organs and *jingluo*. Moreover, it discriminates between thoracic, nutrient and defensive *qi* and that in the various *zang* and *fu* organs and *jingluo*. *Jingluo* can be used to activate the whole and different parts of the body. *Jing*, blood, and clear and mucoid fluid supplies the activity of *qi* in the body with *qi*. Under its command, *zang* and *fu*, *jingluo*, *jing*, blood, and clear and mucoid fluid form a complete entity. *Qi* carries information within the body, and this internal information is manifested outwardly. Mental activity is an even higher expression of basic *qi*. A *qigong* master can direct his genuine *qi* by means of will to various body parts. He can also bring his potential ability into full play to display a kind of immense power.

When the activity of *qi* is in a state of relative equilibrium between yin and yang, the human body is healthy. *Huang Di Nei Jing* says that minor fire (a normal physiological fire) produces *qi*. If yin and yang in the human body are not balanced, or if *qi* in the whole body, or else in the *zang-fu* organs, has lost its normal order, obstructions of different degrees will take place. For instance, dampness, which is one among the six exogenous pathogenic factors, is characterized by yin; it will block and retard *qi* and give rise to such problems as lassitude, debility of the limbs, poor appetite and stuffiness in the chest. Thinking to fortify the body, some make lavish use of such kinds of *qi*-reinforcing and yang-invigorating drugs as hairy antler, ginseng, astragalus, etc., regardless of the users' physical conditions. If the patient does not have the deficiency of yang or lack of *qi*, they will be incapable of sustaining the action of these kinds of drugs, which may inversely induce light-headedness, nervousness, lassitude, and even bleeding from the mouth and nose. *Huang Di Nei Jing* therefore comments about "the strong pathogenic fire which consumes *jing*," namely the hyperfunction of yang which affects the normal operation of *qi*.

The integration of yin and yang is likewise expressed in the ascent and descent, or in the opening and closing, of the body's *qi*. Normally, clear fluid ascends and thick mucoid fluid descends. If this becomes unbalanced, however, if clear yang does not ascend and mucoid yin does not descend, distention of the epigastrium, confusion, general discomfort, and similar symptoms will occur.

The line of reasoning of Chinese drugs regarding *siqi* and *wuwei*, floating and sinking, opening and closing, is to rectify the activity of the body's *qi*. It is therefore necessary to consider the problem of *qi* seriously. In Chinese medical theory, the physique, *qi* and divine spirit are related with *qi* as their center. With little understanding of *qi* and its activity, a profound understanding of the essence and secrets of Chinese medicine is impossible. In its study of the phenomena of life and pathology, from macrodissection to the structure of the molecule, Western medicine pays more attention to individual organs and tissues. However, the study of *qi* and activity of *qi*, which are vital to life, and of the "divine spirit" that is its expression in a higher form, are a field that Western medicine should penetrate more deeply. By now, foreign scientists have gradually become conscious of its importance. For instance, Albert Szent-Györgyi (1893-?), a well-known biophyscist and biochemist, says in his *Electrobiology and Cancer*, "Our body is constructed of many molecules, mainly protein macromolecules. Therefore, it is naturally believed that all biological response must be molecular response, making life into a kind of molecular phenomenon. The charm of biology lies in the extreme ingenuity of its various responses. Therefore, I never believe that these responses are induced by those clumsy macromolecules without participation by smaller, more active and more sensitive units, which could only be the electrons that are non-localized and have high reaction activity." Aren't these smaller, more active and sensitive units closely comparable to the concept of *qi* in Chinese medicine?

At the moment, comparatively rapid progress and significant accomplishments have been made by integrating Chinese and Western medicine in the study of promoting blood flow to eliminate blood stasis, including the study of microcirculation. We expect that this study, especially that made by Xiu Ruijuan, a woman medical expert in China, will contribute to a further scientific understanding of *qi*. This is because Chinese medicine believes that "*qi* is in command of blood," and that "if *qi* circulates, blood will follow; if *qi* is stagnant, blood will silt up." *Qi* and blood are a closely related unity. A profound understanding of blood will advance our understanding of *qi*. At the same time, *qi* in Chinese medicine enjoys a far wider scope. There are, for instance, several varieties of *qi* in *qigong* exercises, in *jingluo*, in the *zang-fu* organs, along with constructive, defensive, thoracic, and genuine *qi*, each having its own peculiar contents and functions. Knowledge of Chinese medicine will promote understanding of the phenomenon of life.

6) Along with *jingluo*, the *zang* and *fu* organs form a holistic relationship. All the channels and collaterals in *jingluo* intersect each other throughout the body: trunks running longitudinally are channels, while collaterals are thready strings running horizontally. They are passages for the circulation of *qi*, blood, and clean and mucoid fluids, and so guarantee the activity of the body's *qi* and facilitate communication from top to bottom and between interior and exterior. As a result, *zangxiang* forms a unified holistic relationship with nature.

The *jingluo* system comprises 12 channels, eight extra channels, 15 collaterals, branches of the 12 channels, musculature of the 12 channels, 12 cutaneous regions, and a countless myriad of tiny branches— the minor collaterals. The 12 channels connect directly with the six *zang*[23] (heart, liver, spleen, lung, kidney and pericadium) and six *fu* organs. They are joined one by one at the head and face, in the trunk, on the four extremities, longitudinally, horizontally, on top and below, in accordance with their yin or yang nature and their superficial or internal localities, thereby constituting the main passages for *qi* and blood circulation and for constructing the interior and defending the exterior. The branches of the 12 channels circulate deep within the body. They begin at the four limbs and enter the internal organs, and come out again at the head and neck; they circulate along with the yin and yang channels. Whether exiting or entering, separating or joining, each is always alternately the interior or the exterior of the other. The musculature of the 12 channels does not enter the *zang-fu* organs, but instead starts from the extremities of the four limbs, travels to the joints, up to the head, neck and face, penetrating the muscles of the various parts of human body and strengthening the connection between the interior and exterior. The eight extra channels include the back midline channel, which governs all the yang channels, and the front midline channel, which connects with all the yin channels. These two channels maintain a relationship with each other and link all the channels. Other extra channels perform a connecting and converging function, like a labyrinth of lakes and marshes which regulate the water of rivers and streams. The body is accordingly a network in which all the extremities can be reached and any part of the body is accessible. *Zangxiang* presents a closely related holistic system related to body parts as well as particular organs. Through *qi* of the channels, the activities of the *zang-fu* organs are connected and regulated with those of *jing*, blood, constructive and defensive *qi*, clear and mucoid body fluid. A set of methods, original and effective, has been formulated in the preventive and therapeutic theories as well as acupuncture, moxibustion, massage and *qigong* therapy of traditional Chinese medicine. They include taking acupoints at relevant and irrelevant channels, at the lower body when illness occurs in the upper body, at the upper body when illness is at the lower, as well as scalp-acupuncture and auriculo-acupuncture....

Acupuncture anesthesia is now starting to replace narcotic in certain Western operations, advancing the application of *jingluo* and acupuncture into a new field and arousing great interest and enthusiasm. When research in anatomical, histological and physiological fields met with failure, Prof. Zhang Xiangtong, a famous Chinese neurologist, carried on his study from a holistic point of view and discovered that acupuncture anesthesia can trigger the hypothalamus to secrete *nephetai*, which acts on the nerves and induces an analgesic affect on a specific locality. His study proves that although acupuncture anesthesia is locally administered, the effect is realized through the body's holistic relationship. Therefore, research into Chinese medicine should begin with a study of the holistic system.

A summary of this chapter offers the following leading principles:

1) The *zangxiang* theory is built on the basis of a holistic relationship. The antagonism and unity of yin and yang and the order of *wuxing* are basic to the study of human physiology and pathology. This theory takes the interrelation between mankind and nature, the interior and exterior of the *zang* and *fu* organs, and between the body and mental activity as a large system of interrelations and interactions. Since every *zang* or *fu* organ is an organic component of a holistic relationship, it can be understood only in terms of this relationship.

2) The *zang* and *fu* organs are a system of interrelated functions in a mutual relationship; this differs from the

system in Western medicine. Of course, the *zang* and *fu* organs are endowed with certain forms and structures; but since the *zangxiang* theory mainly stresses its *qi*, it pays less attention to forms and structures. Similar emphasis should be given in studying traditional Chinese medicine. Because the starting point of Chinese and Western medicine is different, the angle and contents of their study necessarily differ greatly. Neither should maintain that its own cognition is absolute and repudiate the other as absurd; both should instead conduct a comparative study on the basis of theoretical methodology. Each should draw on the strong points of the other and bridge the gulf between the two in order to create a new medical science.

3) In order to recognize human physiology and pathology, traditional Chinese medicine has employed methods of dissection to a certain extent, although such methods have been coarse, simple and shallow. In most cases, its method remains similar to "not opening the black box" in cybernetics. Its recognition of the *zang* and *fu* functions is obtained mainly through the input and output of information. In addition, there might possibly be a self-sensing method called the "reverberating view of inside scene," which to an even greater extent differs from such modern Western methods as dissection, analysis and reduction, and the method of "opening the box". We should draw on others' strong points to make up for our own shortcomings while developing all of our own strong points. By indiscriminately imitating the methods of Western medicine and discarding those of Chinese medicine, we will not learn or advance, and may even be led astray.

Chapter IV

THE *BIANZHENGLUNZHI* THEORY

Genesis

The sciences of medicine and pharmacology have developed as man has; in primitive society, therapeutic practices were closely connected with primitive labor and daily life. In the primitive times, people lived as savages, in caves or in the wilderness, eating birds and raw meat. Under such extremely crude and rough conditions, they were frequently threatened by diseases and wounds, but at that time, they had no knowledge of medicine and medical care. By gathering food, fishing, hunting and raising crops, they gradually learned which vegetables and animals were edible and wholesome and which poisonous and inedible. They also learned which things caused them to vomit or to have diarrhea. In some cases, sick people ate foods which made them feel better, while others might have rubbed tree bark or a particular stone on their body where it ached and found that the pain was thereby relieved. Through accumulated practice and experience, they gradually learned how to utilize certain things to treat their bodies. The simple application of drugs and stone needle acupuncture thus became the embryonic stage of medicine. *Huang Di Nei Jing* states: "In the east of China, diseases were mostly ulcers, for which the stone needle was the best treatment." In ancient times, in areas where the weather was hot and humid, people were liable to be affected with ulcers, and had already learned to use the stone needle to open the ulcer to force out the pus. Shen Nong, founder of agriculture and medicine in the Chinese legend, is said to have tasted a multitude of herbs in China. *Huai Nan Zi*, a book on various natural and social sciences written by Liu An in the Han Dynasty, says, "Shen Nong tasted the flavor of a hundred herbs and the sweetness or bitterness of springs and fountains in order that people would know what they should guard against. He would taste 70 kinds of poison at most in a single day." This account reveals that gathering and farming clans grew vegetables as the principal means of subsistence. Through practice, they came to know about a large variety of herbs and waters, and additionally learned from cases of poisoning.

An interesting story tells how people in the West learned the function of a plant. The tomato, which is very popular today, was first found in the forests of Peru. Seeing its brilliant color, people thought that it was poisonous and were careful not to eat it. It was then grown in the garden as an ornamental plant. This plant was brought back to England by an English duke who toured South America and presented them to Queen Elizabeth in the 16th century. It was called an apple of love in Europe and sent to lovers as a token of affection. Still, generation after generation, no one dared to eat it. About 200 years later, a French painter, fascinated by the splendor of the fruit, decided to take the risk. After writing his will, he ate a tomato and became the first man to have tasted the sweet and sour of the fruit. Only then did the tomato become a delicious dish served at the dining table. Similarly, ancient Chinese dared to risk "tasting 70 poisons in a single day," and succeeded in acquiring knowledge of a broad variety of herbs. As many as 369 kinds of herbal drugs were listed in *Shen Nong Ben Cao* ("Shen Nong's Herbal"), first of its kind in China, which reflect the devotion of Chinese people to science.

Mankind has acquired increasingly more experience

through social practice. Knowledge of diseases in different locations in the body has gradually increased and experience conducting simple heteropathy has accumulated. Inscriptions on bones and tortoise shells unearthed from the Shang Dynasty (c. 16th-11th century B.C.) ruins record terms for headache, otopathy, eye and nose diseases, odontopathy— all reflecting knowledge about diseases.

Following the development of agriculture, during the period of economy based on hunting and animal husbandry, people acquired more information about the shape and internal structure of animals. Deaths and wounds caused by wars between clan tribes, as well as the cruel slaughter of captives, also provided a further opportunity to acquire insight into muscle and bones, the shape of the *zang* and *fu* organs, as well as simple therapeutic methods for curing diseases. In this way mankind accumulated, through long years of study and practice, knowledge of the structure and functions of the human body, and also of diseases, medical care and medicine.

The development from scattered medical experience and knowledge to a medical theory guided by a certain doctrine is a great leap. This "leap" in China began in the pre-Qin era when Chinese society progressed rapidly following the widespread use of iron. The development of culture and thought reached a climax at that time. In philosophy, naive materialism and dialectics— the yin and yang, and *wuxing* theories— were gradually introduced. When this was integrated with what had been learned about the physiology of the *zang* and *fu* organs, along with diseases and their treatment, an academic system based on the theories of yin and yang, *zangxiang* and *bianzhenglunzhi* gradually formed. These theories were constantly formed and revised as time passed. Under their guidance, Chinese medicine and pharmacology gradually passed from the heteropathy of experimental medicine to the theory-guided treatment.

Huang Di Nei Jing is the oldest medical classic in

China today. Its compilation probably began during the Spring and Autumn Period (770-476 B.C.) and the Period of Warring States and was completed during the Qin and Han dynasties. It was the crystallization of the collective wisdom of medical workers and philosophers at that time. *Huang Di Nei Jing* comprehensively explored the theories of yin and yang and the *zang* and *fu* organs. It provided, however, only an embryonic form of the theory of *bianzhenglunzhi*. It was systematically completed by Zhang Zhongjing in his work *Shang Han Za Bing Lun* ("Treatise on Febrile and Miscellaneous Diseases"), in the last years of the Eastern Han Dynasty (25-220). He says in a preface to *Shang Han Lun*:

> I was grieved at the bereavement of my beloved ones in the past and pained by the failure to save unnatural and premature deaths. Therefore, I had been earnestly in quest of ancient teachings and in searching widely for folk prescriptions from all directions. Making use of the nine volumes of *Huang Di Nei Jing* and *Nan Jing*, I compiled *Shang Han Za Bing Lun*, together in a total of 16 volumes. Although the book might fail to cure all diseases, it will help to locate their sources. If what I have collected is consulted, then over half of the troubles could be solved.

In this connection, Zhang clarifies that his idea of *bianzhenglunzhi* came from the widespread practices of people and from the guidance of *Huang Di Nei Jing* and *Nan Jing*. His work also deals with the relationships between various theories of traditional medicine and the development of those theories— from practice to theory and practice again.

Bianzheng and Treatment

Some people take "syndromes" to mean the series of symptoms and signs manifesting diseases. This viewpoint, however, is neither comprehensive nor correct. Of course, *bianzheng* (the differentiation of syndromes) in Chinese medicine begins from a series of symptoms and signs. These only reflect the existence of an illness, however; they do not reveal its cause. No Chinese doctor can really cure diseases if he does not know their causes and fails to master their regularity. Chinese medicine has always opposed treating the head when the head aches or the foot when the foot aches: Rigid heteropathy— administering treatment only in accordance with superficial phenomena— is the frivolous trick of a charlatan. In order to have a comprehensive understanding of the patient's symptoms, differentiation must start with the four methods of diagnosis: observation, auscultation and olfaction, interrogation and pulse-taking.

However, this is only the perceptual stage. Based on this information, the physician must be guided by theory and method to discover the causes and location of the illness, apprehend its nature, and determine its development. Only then can he understand the source and substance of the disease. Therefore, the diagnostic methods used by Chinese medicine include the following features of a disease: the symptoms and signs, the causes— *liuyin* (six external pathogenic factors): wind, cold, summer heat, dampness, dryness and heat; *qiqing* (seven emotions): joy, anger, anxiety, worry, grief, apprehension and fright; and the retention of external pathogens— the site of the disease (external or internal, in which organ), the nature of affections (cold, heat, deficient, excessive, yin, yang) and the developmental tendency and prognosis of the disease. Only after the physician has advanced from initial perceptions to knowledge of the disease will he be able to decide the treating principles, work out correct prescriptions and administer medicine. The following diagram outlines the relationship between symptoms and signs and differentiated syndromes.

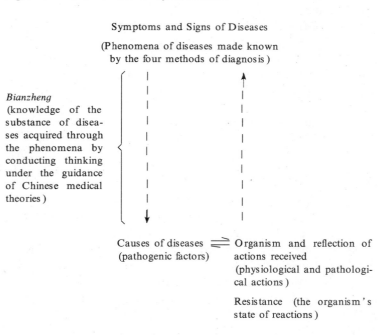

Pathogenic factors, whether originating outside or inside the body, act on organisms and cause them to react differently when they are different. Nevertheless, there is some difference in reactions when the pathogenic factors are the same. The reason is that people are quite different from one another in constitution and surroundings. But they are always reflected in an organism in the form of various symptoms and signs, from which the physician can find the relationship between pathogenic factors and organism and learn about the essence of a disease. Therefore, "differentiated indications" is first taken as the essence of a disease, in order to comprehend the organism's reaction. This method is quite different from the one used in Western medicine in which the essence of a disease is mainly learned about from its pathogenic factors and foci.

Both the Chinese differentiation of "syndrome" and the Western one of "disease", however, require a physician to learn about the essence of a disease from its symptoms and signs; on this point the two are the same. The difference is that Chinese medicine uses traditional theories and methods to tell one symptom from another and form a concept of "syndrome." (Of course, there is a concept of "disease" in Chinese medicine, too.) Western medicine, however, uses its theories and methods to tell one disease from another and has a concept of "disease" of its own. The disease is the same in both Chinese and Western medical sciences. As their methods are different, two concepts— "syndrome" and "disease"— are formed, and two kinds of treatment prepared, one based on the analysis of syndrome and the other on that of disease. Today, integration of these two methods has already helped in curing disease and shortening the course of treatment. One must always remember, however, that both are built on two entirely different theoretical systems; integration is only a bridge on the road to progress. To reach our destination, the internal relationship between differentiating the syndrome and disease must be clarified for the creation of a unified theory.

The *bianzhenglunzhi* theory holds that diseases are caused by the action of pathogenic factors upon organism and the reaction of the latter, and it emphasizes this internal reaction of an organism. *Bianzheng* includes the differentiation of pathological factors in accordance with the eight main syndromes, pathological changes in *zang-fu* organs, and *liujing*, as well as *wei, qi, ying* and *xue* and triple energizer. The basic principle is to discover how the body is reacting to pathological factors. The following is a description of these methods:

1) The differentiation of pathological factors in accordance with the eight main syndromes is the most basic method. It observes symptoms and signs of the pa-

tient through the four methods of diagnosis; and according to the strength or weakness of the constitution, it analyzes and synthesizes the symptoms, the nature of the affection, the depth of the foci of diseases and the organism's reaction. It thereby generalizes the disease into yin or yang, exterior or interior, cold or heat, and deficient or excessive affections in order to differentiate the syndromes. Of the eight syndromes, exterior, excessive and heat affections are yang; interior, deficient and cold affections are yin. Therefore, yin and yang are in control of the other syndromes, and their balance determines the organism's reactions against the diseases.

Because the organism constantly moves and changes, its exterior and interior, cold and heat, deficient and excessive, and yin and yang also change. External problems may develop internally, while interior affections may find an outlet to the exterior. A cold affection, if pent up too long, may change into heat; a heat affection may turn into cold when *qi* is exhausted. A deficient affection may become excessive due to stasis caused by poor circulation and dissolution caused by a functional decline. An excessive affection may become deficient when genuine *qi* is impaired and lost. When yin is impaired, the effect may spread to yang; when yang impaired, the effect may spread to yin. In all cases, the change is determined by the organism's reaction during the development of the disease. Early practitioners summarized the regularities of these changes. For instance, an external affection's entrance into the interior worsens the disease, but when an internal affection leaves, the disease retreats. The change of a cold into a heat affection means a turn for the better, that of a heat affection into a cold one a turn for the worse. Both deficiency and excess are easy to appear. In general, it is favorable for a yin affection to turn to yang, adverse for a yang to turn to yin.

    2) *Bianzheng* according to pathological changes of *zang-fu* organs is based on observations obtained from the four methods of diagnosis. Chinese medicine maintains

that most of diseases are caused by disruptions to the balance of yin and yang and the functions of the *zang-fu* organs. Due to different functions and sequential positions, the pathological reactions of different *zang-fu* organs will also differ. Therefore, which *zang* or *fu* organ is attacked can be diagnosed from the composite reactions revealed by symptoms and signs. For instance, since the lung is in charge of breath and respiration, it dissipates defensive *qi*. When a patient has contracted a cold, he coughs, pants and shivers. A composite analysis, comparison and differentiation will show that these symptoms are a pathological reflection of the defensive system of the lung, which has been invaded by wind and cold and whose defensive yang has been restrained. It is then ascertained to be a symptom-complex of pulmonary invasion by wind and cold. If the patient coughs, sweats or is feverish, thirsty and has a yellow tongue and a rapid pulse, the protracted stasis caused by pathogenic cold has been pent up too long and turned into heat; the symptom-complex has changed into a lung injured by pathogenic heat. In another instance, differentiated syndromes in cardiac diseases, which are commonly seen, include palpitation and slow functional activity caused by a weakened heart or deficient heart yang; restlessness and poor sleep caused by deficient cardiac blood; aphtha, blush and a liability to anger due to strong and excessive cardiac fire; a dark tongue, stuffy chest and cardiac pain caused by cardiac blood stasis; and mental confusion caused by weakened cardiac movement and mania caused by phlegmy fire disturbing the heart. These indications focus on the reactions caused by the disturbance of yin-yang balance and of the functions of the relevant *zang-fu* organs.

3) *Bianzheng* in *liujing*, mentioned in *Shang Han Lun*, is principally a classification of differentiated syndromes of reactions and their changes from one channel to another after the organism's invasion by external pathogenic factors. Typical patterns of syndromes in *liujing* and their principal syndromes are as follows: Weak pulse, strong

pain on top of the head and an aversion to cold are indications of *Taiyang*. Fever over the body, spontaneous sweating, aversion to heat rather than to cold and constipation are syndromes of *Yangming*. Bitter mouth, dry pharynx and larynx, glazed eyes, intermittent fever and chills, stuffy thorax, anorexia, nervousness and liability to vomit are *Shaoyang* syndromes. Full stomach and regurgitating, lack of appetite, diarrhea, occasional stomach aches, constipation are syndromes of *Taiyin*. A faint pulse and drowsiness are syndromes of *Shaoyin*. Heat in the upper organs and cold in the lower organs, coexistence of cold and heat and alternate prevailing of yin and yang are syndromes of *Jueyin*. In all these syndromes, the organism's reaction is the criterion of classification.

Although *bianzheng* in *liujing* is a way to differentiate external indications, its basic theory still derives from the reactions induced by the interaction between the pathological factors and the organism. Therefore, internal diseases with the symptoms described above may likewise be treated by the methods, prescriptions and medicine in *Shang Han Lun*. The same principle holds for the applied therapy of differentiated syndromes of *wei, qi, ying* and *xue*, as well as for those in triple energizer.

4) The differentiation of indications of *wei, qi, ying* and *xue* represents the four stages in the development of acute febrile diseases. The invasion of the pathogen begins with the surface of the *wei* system, when the pathological focus is the lung, skin and the tongue. The principal symptoms are slight intolerance to wind and cold, fever, intolerable thirst, uncomfortable throat and a floating pulse. The pathogen then enters the *qi* system focusing on the lung or thorax, stomach and intestines, or the liver and gallbladder. The principal symptoms are tolerance of cold but aversion to heat, thirst, large and excessive pulse. The disease then enters the third, or nutrient, phase when the focus is the heart and pericardium, and the principal symptoms are hemorrhage, partial loss of

consciousness, and a red tongue. It finally enters the *xue* system in the liver and kidney, showing an arbitrary blood flow forced by heat. Since the liver does not hold blood, it is forced to bleed, and when the pathogenic heat exhausts the blood the muscles are not nourished. This is liable to induce hepatic wind and tight muscles and tendons, giving vent to convulsion and tics. The tongue also turns red. These are the syndromes of the blood phase.

The development of a disease in the four systems is much like that of an acute infectious disease. When infectious agents invade, the body will react in an all-round way at first. Symptoms of fever, aversion to cold, and some symptoms in the upper respiratory tract appear, the *wei* system is diseased. When the agents breed further, diffuse and aggravate the body with their toxicity, the organism mobilizes a greater resistant force to combat them. Stronger reactions like extreme heat and thirst, profuse sweating, asthma, a large pulse and other symptoms then set in. They are similar to syndromes of the *qi* system. If a stronger resistance fails to get rid of the pathogens, either, the disease then goes into the *ying* and *xue* systems with the appearance of a series of toxin symptoms, like septicemia or bacterial virus, interfering with the nervous system.

There are certain therapeutic rules about changes in the four stages of a disease. Ye Tianshi (1667-1746), a specialist in febrile diseases, pointed out that diaphoresis may be used when the pathogen enters the *wei* system, and only when it enters the *qi* system can the febrifugal method be used, and it may be used, too, when the *ying* system becomes infected. Blood will be exhausted and irritated, and there is every need to cool and disperse blood when the disease enters the *xue* system. It is obvious that the classification of patterns of syndromes and therapeutic principles are considered mainly from the viewpoint of the organism's reaction.

5) *Bianzheng* in triple energizer is classified in accordance with a concept of triple energizer in *Huang Di*

Nei Jing and based on the three stages of acute febrile disease, and is therefore used in the treatment of that disease caused by dampness and heat. Dampness is a yin pathogen liable to damage the yin fluid, so the disease caused by dampness and heat generally exists somewhere between the *wei* and *ying* systems. Since its heat co-exists with dampness, it is difficult to tell cold from heat on the one hand and determine whether it is in the *wei* system or the *qi* one. Dampness is heavy and turbid and tends to descend. Chinese medicine maintains that triple energizer functions as a passage of the activity of *qi* and water. Therefore, in his work *Wen Bing Tiao Bian* ("Detailed Analysis of Epidemic Febrile Diseases"), Wu Tang (1758-1836) accordingly adopted the classification of triple energizer. Syndromes of the upper energizer include mild fever pathogen which attacks upward and first invades the lung but then moves to the pericardium. The lung is in charge of *qi* and belongs to the *wei* system; the heart is in charge of blood and belongs to the *ying* system. The principal symptoms of pulmonary invasion by mild fever pathogen are fever with a slight intolerance to cold, headache, spontaneous sweating, slight thirst and rapid external pulse. Those of pericardial invasion include high fever (specially at night), loss of consciousness, delirium, nervousness and sleepless, thirst but a disinclination to drink and a reddish purple tongue.

Syndromes of the middle energizer affect the three channels of the spleen, the stomach and the large intestine. When a pathogen enters the middle energizer and desiccates it, the principal symptoms are fever, abnormal aversion to heat but not to cold, high fever in the afternoons with a flushed face and red eyes, dull voice and heavy respiration, constipation, astringent urine, a yellow tongue and syndromes of excessive heat in the stomach and intestines. If the disease enters the middle energizer and causes dampness, then the bodily heat will not dissipate and there will be stuffiness in the chest, nausea and a tendency to vomit, heavy body and tired limbs, glossy tongue and oft pulse and such symptoms as indissolubility of the spleen.

Syndromes of the lower energizer are protracted mild fever pathogen, which exhausts and hurts hepatic and renal yin. The principal symptoms are hot body and red face, hot palms and soles, dry mouth with thirst, dry lips, lassitude, anxiety and sleeplessness. If a deficient wind moves internally, the hands and feet cramp or spasm, the limbs numb and the heart trembles. Obviously, syndrome differentiation in triple energizer starts from the action exerted by the pathogenic factors of mild or humid heat, and from the organism's reaction to that stimulus.

The various methods of *bianzheng* observe the substance and regularities of diseases from different viewpoints and are used to guide clinical practice. In the past, in fact there were controversies between the school of classic prescriptions and the school of acute febrile diseases. It is irreproachable for each to express his own view and contend with others, drawing on others' strengths to make up for one's own weaknesses. If one sticks only to his own view and repudiates anything alien, refusing to respect and learn from others, his actions are incompatible with the fundamental principle of traditional medicine.

In differentiating diseases, Western medicine also pays attention to the organism's reaction, because symptoms and signs help them to have some understanding of a disease. However, even though there are morphological classifications and functional classifications of diseases in Western medicine, its major trend is towards the classification of the causes of diseases. It seeks to recognize the nature and regularities of diseases from their causes. Therefore, Western medicine adopts the contra-cause treatment; other types of treatment, like supporting treatment and heteropathy, are only used as auxiliary means. For instance, Western medicine maintains that pulmonary tuberculosis is induced by the invasion of the lungs by the

the tubercle bacillus, and thus it administers antituberculous drugs to annihilate the bacillus. Although patients A, B, C, and D are different human beings, the causes of their diseases are the same, despite the different expressions of their symptoms. The principal therapeutic methods adopted by Western medicine are the same, too; as a result, Western medicine has no need to differentiate the symptoms.

The Chinese method, however, focuses on the organism's reaction, not on the pathogens causing the disease, so it seldom uses the same prescriptions to deal with tubercle bacilli. Patients A, B, C and D are different from one another in constitution, and their surroundings and other conditions are not the same, so they can hardly make identical reactions to the bacilli and present the same symptoms. Some may have a cough with little phlegm, low fever in afternoons, heat in the chest, palms and soles, a dry mouth, red cheeks, nervousness and insomnia, night sweating, and tight and rapid pulse. Such syndromes are attributable to the deficiency of yin in the lung and kidney in Chinese medicine. Other tuberculars may have a cough with much phlegm, little strength, loss of appetite, a feeble voice, pale face, and abnormal pulse, due to the deficiency of yang in the lung and kidney. Taking these into account, the doctor will prepare different prescriptions for the two types of patients, giving medicine for yin and *qi* to the former but medicine to support yang in the spleen and lung to the latter. In treating tuberculosis, a Chinese doctor usually uses such kinds of drugs as *Radix Stemonae* and *Spica Prunellae* to suppress tubercle bacilli. Its aim is to regulate the relationship between yin and yang in the organism in order to help it regain the balance and fight against the disease. Comparing these two instances, we can see that the invasion of the lungs by tubercle bacilli is the cause of death common to all tuberculars, but other factors such as constitution and surroundings should also be taken into consideration. This has been realized by some doctors of

Western medicine. In their opinion, etiology has its own limitations because constitution, surroundings and psychology and society and other factors are often neglected in the treatment of diseases, especially of cardiovascular diseases, cancer and psychosis. To change this situation, many Western medical specialists are beginning to pay attention to theories about diseases and constitutions and to the study of the body's reactions towards various stimulations and the various patterns of these reactions.

All this shows that both "disease" and "man" should be dealt with in the treatment of diseases. Sun Simiao (581-682) says in his *Qian Jin Yao Fang* ("Prescriptions Worth a Thousand Gold") says: "A good physician usually pays attention to the prevention of diseases in a vast piece of land, a mediocre physician tries to learn about the general conditions of a patient while giving medical treatment, but a poor physician treats only the disease itself to the neglect of other conditions." If attention is focused merely on treating the "disease," while forgetting the "man," it might often happen that although the cause is eliminated, the man still remains in a very inharmonious state of exhaustion or discomfort. It might even happen that while the illness in question has been brought under control, certain new diseases might enter. On the other hand, if attention is focused merely on treating the organism of "man," while neglecting the cause of the disease, it may often happen that the patient's symptoms have improved, but the cause has not been completely eliminated, and the trouble is still lurking. Therefore, the aim of our new medical science is to learn about both the universality and particularity of a disease, and try to cure both the disease and man.

A further point should be made clear. In treating infectious diseases, Chinese medicine starts with the organism's reaction to readjust the balance between yin and yang and the order of the body's organs. The question then arises: Is it possible to kill the microorganisms and get rid of the disease completely? Can we say that Chinese medicine only cures the "symptoms," but not the "disease"? To answer this question, we must first review the Chinese medical principle of treatment. The following assertions from *Huang Di Nei Jing* are very meaningful: "Where the pathogenic factors converge, genuine *qi* is certainly deficient. If genuine *qi* exists inside, exogenous pathogenic factors will not invade. If the interior and exterior of the body are in accord, pathogenic factors can do no harm." That is, when pathogenic microorganisms cause diseases due to the body's deficiency and weakness and its little resistance, it is possible for pathogenic factors to further deprive the organism of its balance and order, thus giving rise to diseases. Facts have proven that numerous pathogenic microorganisms exist on the skin, inside the oral cavity, in the intestines, and nearly everywhere in the normal human body. Microbiology tells us that there are 10^{13} cells in the body of an adult. Since a man lives in a natural environment, his body surface and cavities contain some 10^{14} microorganisms, many of them pathogenic. Living practice has shown that these microorganisms will not cause diseases when the organism is healthy. Only when the resistance breaks down— due to overfatigue, poor nutrition, vile natural environment— and the relative equilibrium and the order suffer impairment, can they induce diseases. The attack of disease is therefore the process of struggle between genuine *qi* and pathogenic factors. On the one hand, such factors can further aggravate the disharmony between yin and yang and accelerate disease development; on the other, an organism attempts to combat pathogenic factors. During invasion, it tries to restore the relative equilibrium between yin and yang and the body's order in order to restore its resistance and defeat the pathogens. Many diseases are cured without the help of drugs because the organism has mobilized its resistance and succeeded in defeating them. Even Louis Pasteur (1822-1895), a French scientist who devoted his life to the study of microorganisms, said before his death: "After all, a microorganism is nothing, as everything is an organism." The fundamental factor determining health or illness is internal— genuine qi but not external— pathogenic factors. In the two million years since mankind's coming into the world, more than 99 percent of the time was spent with no knowledge of medicine. In the long past, mankind had constantly suffered from attacks by pathogenic microorganisms, which existed long before the advent of mankind. Human survival certainly depends not only on antiseptic drugs but also on organic resistance. Since the development of a disease is a struggle between body resistance and pathogenic factors, there are two methods available in Chinese medicine. One is to enhance body resistance against pathogenic factors and the other is to dispel pathogenic factors to get rid of the disease.

Traditional Chinese medicine holds that medical treatment should be given after making an overall analysis of the disease and grasping the main part of it. In dealing with certain infectious diseases, Chinese medicine often bases its own principle of treatment on the organism's reaction to the infectious microorganisms; in rendering treatment, prescriptions sometimes contain herbs which resist the pathogens. There are also cases, however, when no drug containing anti-pathogenic microorganisms is used and yet similar results are obtained. This is because the balance between yin and yang and the body's order are regulated, and resistance mobilized and the pathogens suppressed and eliminated.

Present medical practice also holds that the internal stability of an organism is a prerequisite for keeping fit. When pathogenic factors disturb this stability, disease will not attack if the organism is strong enough to readjust the affected functions in time, and if it can rapidly eliminate pathogenic factors, rectify the abnormal changes and restore stability. If it does attack, convalescence will soon begin. Therefore, the more stable the body, the less liable it is to disturbance by pathogenic factors. That means almost the same as what is said in *Huang Di Nei Jing*. "If genuine qi exists inside, exogenous pathogenic factors will be warded off." On the contrary, if the organism is weak, the stability will be easily destroyed by external factors; the organism can be hardly repaired after it is destroyed, and disease will set in. That has almost the same meaning as the sentence that "where the pathogenic factors converge, genuine qi is deficient."

There are two ways to increase the organism's stability. One is to strengthen the functions and systems of important organs, eliminate the pathogenic factors, and readjust the systems if necessary. The other is to inhibit the organism's reaction to the pathogenic irritation in order to mitigate the extent of the destruction. If the pathogenic factors have already damaged the organism to the point that it would be difficult to restore it if the pathogens were not eliminated, then measures should be taken to dispel the disease. This agrees with Chinese medicine's support of genuine qi and the elimination of pathogenic factors.

Tremendous progress has been made in the development of immunology in recent years. The body's immunocompetence is threefold: defense, self-stability and surveillance. If these three functions are normal, the body will remain balanced, resist infection, eliminate noxious substances and inhibit changes in the cells. If the immunocompetence is especially high or low, the organism is likely to form an unbalanced state, which is in turn liable to induce allergies, autoimmune diseases and neoplasm. Although the immunocompetence can be classified into these three phases, their functions and principles are basically identical; they are all responses to the interactions between the organism and the xenogenic macromolecules— the antigenic substances like bacteria and their toxins which have entered the body. These responses produce antibodies and related immune factors which maintain stability. Recently, there have been many reports about the use of drugs which have no antiseptic function but are very therapeutic in curing bacterial diseases. This is because these kinds of drugs mobilize the body's immunocompetence and thus resist infection. Clinical observation finds that the phagocitic index of macrophagocytes of patients with chronic bronchitis and cervical cancer increases conspicuously after they have been treated by supporting genuine *qi* and nourishing the body. Certain cancer patients with low conversion rates of protolymphocyte, after taking the kinds of drugs that nourish yin and tonify genuine *qi* for two months, have their immunity level elevated. Others with a low level of immunity also have increased immunity after treatment with different prescriptions that help support genuine *qi*. To strengthen immunocompetence is to strengthen resistance. For this reason Chinese medicine often adopts a reinforcing method to treat chronic inflammation and retrograde diseases.

Practice has proven that acupuncture and moxibustion can cure such infectious diseases as bacillary dysentery, malaria, hepatitis, leptospirosis, epidemic hemorrhagic fever and pulmonary tuberculosis. The treatment is principally that of tonifying and purgation, which harmonize genuine *qi* and blood, readjust yin and yang and promote resistance against diseases. The Army No. 202 Hospital of Shenyang Military Region administered acupuncture to 1,383 cases of acute bacillary dysentery, the average hospitalization being 5.4 days. Acupuncture acupoints *tianshu, hegu, zusanli* and others were given needles. A total of 1,264 cases (91.4 per cent of total patients) were cured. This is also related to the strengthening of the body's immunocompetence.

According to the No 12,1974 issue of *The Journal of Medicine in Shanxi*, the kinds of drugs for the promotion of blood circulation by promoting blood stasis have a two-way regulating action on the immune system, which decreases the formation of antibodies (therefore preventing the recurrence of the ABO-type neonatal hemolysis), and also elevates the immunocompetence to a certain degree. Other findings from experiments performed by many medical units: yang-tonifying drugs like *Cortex Cinnamomi*, *Rhizoma Curculiginis*, *Semen Cuscutae*, *Herba Cynomorii* and *Rhizoma Polygonati* may promote the rapid formation of antibodies, those for the tonification of *qi* like *Radix Astragali*, *Radix Codonopsis Pilosulae* and *Ganoderma Lucidum* have a similar or even greater effect than that of BCG vaccine in promoting the engulfing plasma proteins of the reticuloendothelial system in small white rabbits, and those for the nourishing of yin such as *Carapax Trionycis*, *Radix Scrophulariae*, *Radix Asparagi*, *Radix Ophiopogonis* and *Radix Glehniae* prolong the existence of antibodies.

As it is, world problems can often be solved through many different ways. Molds in a moist room can be killed by sprinkling antimycin drug, and the problem can also be solved by opening the windows and doors to let in sunshine and ventilate the room, thus changing it from a moist into a dry one. The growth and propagation of microbes are related to the environmental conditions, and a change in the latter will promote changes in them. Since pathogenic microbes live within the body, adjustment and change of the conditions of the organism to change the internal and external environment of microbes will naturally produce corresponding effects on pathogenic microbes. Therefore, it is understandable that a complete recovery from infectious diseases produced by pathogenic microbes is entirely possible.

The application of specific drugs against specific germs is not effective when the functions of an organism are weak or unbalanced because of a protracted illness. Often the condition cannot be in control for a long time. This is because the relationship between the organism and the drugs are only external causes or conditions, while organism is the internal cause or the fundamental ground, and external causes will be operative only through the action of internal causes. Now that the function of organism has already become very weak, the drugs, being the exogenous causes, will be difficult to be operative. At this point, the application of the Chinese medical method of *bianzhenglunzhi* will fix its attention on endogenous causes, on adjusting the balance of yin and yang, and restoring the order of the *zang-fu* organs, and will often have a good curative effect.

In summary, the theory of *bianzhenglunzhi* maintains that "where pathogenic factors converge, genuine *qi* is certainly insubstantial." Because the organism is unstable and aggravated by pathogenic factors, the relative equilibrium between yin and yang and the order of the *zang-fu* organs are further impaired, resulting in an attack of the disease. Effected by pathogens and organism, reaction will vary in the form of symptoms and signs, depending on constitution, surroundings, season and climate. The guiding ideology of traditional Chinese medicine in this area is threefold: using the principle "carefully scrutinizing the sites of yin and yang" and balancing them; investigating the cause of the imbalance between yin and yang and the disorder of the *zang-fu* organs, by studying the yin and yang, exterior and interior, cold and heat, deficient and excessive as guiding principles, and using measures such as medicdation, acupuncture and moxibustion, massage, and therapeutic exercises. In this way, balance and health will be gradually restored, and the resistance and strength of the organism will be rebuilt. The invasion of disease will thus be overcome, resistance enhanced, and pathogenic factors eliminated and health regained. This method complies with the dialectical teaching that endogenous causes are the base, exogenous causes are the conditions, and the latter operate only through the action of the former. These concepts have moreover been gradually witnessed by such modern medical developments as immunology, and contain rich scientific methods and therapeutic effects.

Endogenous causes are the principal ones, but under certain conditions, strong external causes can also unexpectedly injure the body and cause diseases. Therefore, attention should be given to pathogenic factors while laying emphasis on internal causes.

Scrutinizing Syndromes to Search for the Cause of Disease

There is a great difference between Chinese and Western medicine in recognizing the cause of disease. Treatment in Western medicine is mainly based on the causes; it maintains that there is a lineal relationship between each corresponding casual pair of pathogenic factors and diseases, and that the cause of disease determines their substance. Beginning with the early study of bacteriology by Louis Pasteur and Robert Koch (1843-1910), medical science has developed rapidly. As mentioned, the methodology of Western medicine is based principally on dissection, analysis and reduction, and opening the black box. The development of modern sciences has pushed Western medicine to rely more on examination by means of physics, chemistry, biochemistry, physiology and pathological anatomy to search for the causes of disease, such as pathogenic microorganism, water and salt metabolism, cytomorphosis, neurohumoral regulation, body fluid and other factors. That is why Western medicine depends more on laboratory examination and analysis than symptoms and signs for final diagnosis. It is consequently possible to pay attention only to diseases or their causes and neglect the patient himself. Because of this, the patient's emotional, spiritual and mental side is often neglected in favor of the disease diagnosis. The development of science and technology has provided medical science with powerful tools, but it prompts some physicians to rely too much on laboratory reports while neglecting relatively the importance of the thought in differentiating the disease. This tendency should be avoided.

Chinese medicine was formed and developed under the conditions peculiar to ancient Chinese society. At that time, it was incapable of employing modern scientific methods and so Chinese etiology began by "scrutinizing syndromes to search for the cause of disease." The relationship of cause and effect traces the cause from the results; *bianzheng* stresses mainly the organism's reaction to the cause, which is in conformity with the fact the black box is opened to recognize a disease is widely used in Chinese medicine.

There are three types of pathogenic factors according to Chinese medicine: exogenous, endogenous and non-exo-endogenous. The exogenous pathogenic factors comprise wind, cold, summer heat, dampness, dryness and fire and the epidemic noxious atmosphere. The endogenous factors include joy, anger, anxiety, worry, grief, apprehension and fright. Non-exo-endogenous factors are pathologic manifestations caused by such pathogens as rotting food, accumulated phlegm and fluid, and blood stasis. The last two categories cause diseases which are either brought about by the organism itself when suffering from emotional stimuli, or else induced by pathological products. Most of the causes of these diseases reside within the organism.

Let us start with the exogenous factors. Wind, cold, summer heat, dampness, dryness and fire are originally the six kinds of seasonal climate. The normal climate is called *liuqi*. If the climate becomes abnormal and the body cannot adjust, if it brings about an abnormality in the organism's yin and yang, or if it interrupts the body's stabilized order and reduces the resistance, a disease will be induced and *liuyin* (six pathogenic factors) will appear. *Liuqi* may also include the factors liable to propagate certain pathogenic microorganisms under particular climatic conditions. Thus the relationship between diseases and seasons can be seen from the fact that diseases caused by the pathogenic wind occur more frequently in spring, that those caused by the pathogenic heat occur more often in summer. Likewise, those caused by the pathogenic dryness-fire usually appear in autumn and those caused by the pathogenic cold in winter. Is it possible to locate the pathogenic microorganism of these external factors under a microscope, as Western physicians do? Chinese epidemiology and parasitosis are also conscious of the trouble caused by pathogenic microorganisms or bacterial parasites. It is not, however, from this point of view, that Chinese medicine has established its concept of *liuqi*. Instead, it is after a study of the relationship between the features of *liuyin* and those of the organism's reaction that people have come to know something about *liuyin*. Following are the symptoms of *liuyin* and man's understanding of its nature.

Wind: Wind is a yang pathogenic factor. It injures by means of opening and reducing nature. It attacks the skin, the exterior and upper portion of the human body, and thus usually causes sweating, aversion to wind and headache. The nature of wind is to move and change; therefore its onset is acute and its dissipation quick. The site of attack is difficult to predict and rather capricious. Because wind is predominantly mobile, the symptoms usually include vertigo, shivering, convulsion and opisthotonos.

Cold: Cold is a yin pathogenic factor which can injure yang-*qi*. When cold impairs yang of *qi* in the *wei* system, the body becomes averse to cold. When it impairs yang of the *zang-fu* organs, the symptoms are watery diarrhea, limpid urine and long urination, retching and vomiting of water, dilute phlegm and saliva, cold body and chilly limbs. Cold congeals, stagnates and is prone to cause pain. It coagulates *qi* and blood and blocks their flow; this too causes pain. Therefore, when cold injures the nutrient and defense systems, the body feels pain. If the cold attacks the stomach and intestines directly, the gastral cavity convulses in pain. Cold tends to collect and withdraw. When it is inside the skin and hairs, or in the juncture of the skin and muscles, it makes the pores contract and shrink. Then yang of defensive *qi* becomes blocked and depressed, and the body becomes averse to cold, having fever but no sweating and tense pulsation. When cold penetrates *jingluo*, the muscles and tendons cramp.

Summer heat: Summer heat is a yang pathogenic factor. Since its nature is flaming heat, those who suffer from summer heat have a fever as high as burning charcoal. It ascends and disperses, consumes *qi* and impairs body fluid, causing the juncture of the skin and muscles to evaporate and sweat profusely. When the body is open and reduces too much, it becomes dehydrated, there is thirst, and urine is sparse and red. A strong pathogenic fire consumes *qi*, causing shortness of breath, weakness and a large but insubstantial pulsation. The patient feels suffocated and deranged or may even fall into a coma. Summer heat is often accompanied by dampness. In the summer, the weather is hot but the land is humid and people live in an interchanging atmosphere; and as a result, most summer-heat diseases are accompanied by humid pathogenic complications.

Dampness: Dampness is a yin pathogenic factor that tends to injure yang-*qi* and block the function of *qi*. If dampness impairs the splenic yang, appetite is deceased. If it obstructs the normal flow of *qi*, the chest will sense stuffiness, and it will cause vomiting and loose and uncomfortable bowels; urine will be scant and the pulse soft. Dampness is heavy and turbid. If it remains in the upper part of the body and lucid yang is obstructed from ascending, severe headache ensues and the voice becomes hoarse and raspy. If it is retained in the joints, the limbs become heavy and difficult to raise and move. Dampness is also adhesive and stagnant. For instance, the coating of the tongue will be thick and greasy, stools filthy and turbid, sweat sticky and stagnant, and urine astringent and urination difficult. Most secretions will be greasy and turbid like leukorrhea and gonorrhea. Diseases caused by dampness are frequent and hard to cure.

Dryness: Dryness is liable to hurt body fluid, thus affecting lips, nose, pharynx and skin. Since the lung is in charge of the circulation and readjustment of fluid, and the stomach is the reservoir of water and food, dryness will mostly hurt these organs. If the lung is dry, a dry cough with phlegm or blood; if the stomach is dry, there is thirst and loss of appetite.

Fire: Fire is the utmost heat. Its nature is flaming and ascending, thereby causing fever, aversion to heat, nervousness, uneasiness, flushed face and ears, red tongue with yellow coating, red urine and rapid pulse. When cardiac fire flares up and ascends, the mouth and tongue are blistered; when it erupts in the stomach, the throat and gums swell; when in the liver, the eyes are red and the head aches. Fire is impetuous and liable to burn up fluid; illness caused by fire is consequently acute and capricious. For instance, with a unusually high fever, convulsion and loss of normal mental activity occur. When the body fluid is scorched, the patient is thirsty and anxious to drink cold beverages, the tongue is hot and the throat dry, while the urine and stools are dry and constipated. Because fire radiates heat, it often causes hemorrhages. (Some physicians maintain that there is no such atmospheric energy as fire, that fire is only the extreme of "heat." Moreover, they claim that the fire syndrome is actually transmuted from the other five pathogenic factors. Consequently, they maintain that fire should not be listed as one of the six pathogenic factors. Although this assertion is not without ground, we have kept the old concept of *liuyin* because it is traditional.)

Judging from what is said above, we can see that the theory of *liuyin* has something to do with those of yin and yang, *wuxing* and *zangxiang*, and that according to this theory, the relationship between climate and disease is learned about in the light of that between the nature and the *zang-fu* organs. Whenever *liuqi* becomes abnormal, yin and yang will be affected— deficient or excessive, and different symptoms will appear. For instance, wind, summer heat, dryness and fire are regarded as yang pathogenic factors, while dampness and cold are yin. Through years of practice, Chinese physicians have mastered the inner link of an organism with nature, and the symptoms and causes of diseases, which provides scientific basis for Chinese medicine. This procedure has proved quite effective. One day, a middle-aged man came to see me. He complained of depression, weakness, fatigue and a headache and fever. His skin was found to be yellow and turbid, his chest stuffy and his abdomen distended. He was also nauseated but could not vomit. It was already summer, yet he was still wearing warm clothes. His pulse was soft and his tongue was greasy. He had been in hospital for two months but no correct diagnosis had been formed on his disease, so he came to ask me for help. An examination showed an obstruction of *qi* caused by dampness and turbidity. Then prescriptions were prepared to eliminate dampness, and he felt better very soon.

To diagnose a disease by the reaction of the entire organism is more comprehensive and more helpful in mobilizing the organism's resistance. The body's internal and external surroundings are extremely complicated. There are several kinds of pathogenic factors in many cases, and the causes exist both outside and inside. Looking for the causes, a doctor may take the interaction of many factors and variables before deciding upon an effective plan for treatment. Take encephalitis B for instance. It broke out in the north China city of Shijiazhuang in 1954. The weather was then quite hot, and indications on the patients showed vigorous fire, loss of consciousness and some other symptoms typical of sthenic fever. To treat this disease, doctors of traditional Chinese medicine were called to help with work. They adopted the decoction *baihutang*[24], a kind of drug used to cure sthenic fever, to serve as a a kind of medicine to reduce fever and remove toxic substances. The decoction was administered subject to minor readjustments of ingredients and dosages according to conditions, and good results were gained.

That disease broke out in Beijing a year later, where the weather had been cloudy and drizzly for days on end. The patients had fever, congestion, and were delirious. They suffered from a damp-heat syndrome. Doctors worked out the same prescriptions as they had done in Shijiazhuang a year before, but without avail. Satisfactory results were achieved after prescriptions were changed to lower the fever and the body's dampness. Etiologically, the pathogenic factor of encephalitis B is the encephalitis B virus, so the disease in both Shijiazhuang and Beijing was the same. However, since each city had its own climate, and each patient had his own constitution and reaction to the virus, symptoms and treatment were not the same all the time. The Chinese medical theory on it is in conformity with dialectics and systematics.

Traditional Methods of Diagnosing Symptoms

Traditional Chinese diagnostics possess an original style.

In addition to vision, palpation, percussion and auscultation, there are more methods to be used in Western medicine such as physical diagnosis, chemical tests, bacterial examination, bio-chemical examination, biopsy, and internal exploration through laparotomy (thoracotomy, craniotomy), which help open the black box. That is not the case with traditional Chinese medicine in which only such methods as observation, auscultation and olfaction, interrogation, and pulse-taking and palpation are used. These do not open the black box, but instead identify diseases on the basis of different symptoms. Observation means looking at the patient's facial expression, complexion, and physical build, as well as changes in color and qualities of secretion and reduction. Auscultation and olfaction mean listening to changes in the sound of the patient's voice and breath, and smells the changes in the odor of secretion and discharge from the body. Interrogation refers to an inquiry into the history, attack, development and changes of the disease, along with its treatment and the patient's account of the symptoms. Palpation and pulse-taking comprises touching, pushing and pressing the sites of the illness and its effects. Information about the changes of these symptoms and signs are likewise used as a means of diagnosis. With these methods, a doctor will be able to have a good survey of the disease. However, what he has learned about the disease is just at the perceptual stage of cognition; he has to make an analysis before having a diagnosis of the disease. The correct thinking methods are going from the outside to the inside, proceeding from the one to the other, discarding the dross and selecting the essential and eliminating the false and retaining the true.

Going from the outside to the inside: This means learning about the essence of a thing through its various appearances. The *zangxiang* theory, which asserts that *zang* hides inside but manifests itself outside, is a concept that studies the relationship between the outside of the body and its inner *zang-fu* organs. The differentiation of syndromes according to the eight guiding principles— yin and yang, outside and inside, heat and cold, and deficiency and excess— makes very concrete and detailed descriptions of the interior and exterior images, pointing out which is attributable to which principle. The differentiation of syndromes in accordance with the *liujing* theory and the various syndromes in the *wei, qi, ying* and *xue* systems also provides a means for a doctor to find out the nature of a disease. When finding through observation that the patient coughs with short breath and pale complexion, a doctor would attribute these symptoms to the deficiency of *qi* in the lung; when perceiving a putrid smell from the patient's mouth and noting a thick yellow tongue, he would associate the symptoms with a possible gastric dyspesia; when being told of continual abdominal pain and the need for warmth and pressure, he would consider the cold of deficiency type in the middle and lower energizers;, when finding a superficial pulse, he would suggest that the illness is superficial; and when listening at certain acupoints on the back along the *Taiyang* channel and sensing something different, he would think of an illness in the corresponding *zang* or *fu* organs. These examples show that the theory of rendering treatment according to differentiating syndromes in traditional Chinese medicine guides the physicians in analyzing and synthesizing while they apply those methods of diagnosis, the various kinds of symptoms and signs and proceed from the outside to the inside to discover the essence of diseases from their symptoms.

Proceeding from the one to the other: This notes the relationship between one thing and another thing on the one hand and between one process and another on the other. It is only when we link one thing with others around it can we learn more about it. Emphasis has been laid on the combination of the four methods of diagnosis in Chinese medicine, and the development of a disease and its various symptoms and signs should be taken into account together to find its causes. Take fever for instance. If it is accompanied by symptoms and signs different from person to person, different diseases are contracted. Thus, if fever comes together with a heavy aversion to cold, pain all over the body and superficial pulse, it is usually caused by cold and wind; if fever appears together with a mild aversion to cold, cough, thirst, yellow tongue and rapid pulse, it indicates invasion of the lung by wind and heat; if fever exists with aversion to wind, sweating, tired and heavy limbs, arthritis, difficult movements, stuffy chest and lack of appetite, and soft and slow pulse, it is a sign of a joint invasion by mutually antagonistic wind and dampness; if fever appears with alternate spells of chills, bitter mouth, dry throat, glazed eyes, dysphoria, nausea, distressing fullness in the chest and tight pulse, it indicates a syndrome at the *Shaoyang* channel; if fever arises with dysphoria, loss of consciousness and delirium, dark red tongue, and subcutaneous hemorrhages or bleeding, it suggests that heat is attacking the *ying* and *wei* systems; if a high fever arrives with a frenzied spirit, scaly dry skin, dark gray complexion, thirst but aversion to drink, involuntary urination, and an irregular, deep or tight pulse, it is a syndrome of heat caused by the stagnancy of blood; and if fever is accompanied by a full and stuffy abdominal cavity, nausea, acid regurgitation and fetid belching, yellow tongue and slippery pulse, it is an indication of fever due to spoiled food....

It is therefore clear that fever may have different syndromes under different circumstances. The four methods of diagnosis are accordingly interrelated and indispensable. This is especially true with certain complicated cases which should be treated in the light of other symptoms and signs, willpower and emotion, living surroundings, climate, the history of the disease and the process of treatment. It is after studying the various relationships that a more accurate and correct diagnosis can be made.

Proceeding from one to the other also comprises the transmission, metamorphosis and prognosis of the disease. For instance, an attack of cold on the *Shaoyang* channel produces alternate spells of fever and chills, bitter mouth and parched throat, loss of appetite, dysphoria and nausea. The symptoms of cold and heat indicate that exogenous factors have not yet been completely removed; the others show that the disease is moving toward the interior and will affect the digestive system. During the development of epidemic febrile diseases, if only the tongue has turned red and purple, even though symptoms of *wei* and *qi* systems have not yet disappeared, the diseases are invading the *ying* system. It is pointed out in *Jin Kui Yao Lue* that hepatic diseases are liable to hurt the spleen and stomach. Therefore physicians are told, "When diagnosing a hepatic disease and knowing that it will pass on to the spleen, the spleen should be first made excessive." This is the law governing the development of a disease; by keeping it in mind, the physician will be able to predict future changes at the initial stage of treatment so as to nip the trouble in the bud.

Discarding the dross and selecting the essence: This points to the main contradiction, something that will always play a key role. At the time of diagnosis, the physician may find several dozen symptoms and signs. If he regards them equally, ignoring their individual roles, he will be looking through a kaleidoscope without knowing how to make a diagnosis. Consequently, traditional Chinese medicine teaches one to recognize the principal symptom to discover the root of the disease. Only some symptoms are part of the principal symptom; the others are not directly related, but instead are adjutant or secondary symptoms. Epitomic syndromes, for example, are briefly postulated for syndrome-complex in *liujing* in *Shang Han Lun*. That may be regarded as a good example of the method of discarding the dross and retaining the essence. Take the syndrome of *Taiyang* for instance. It has such symptoms as fever, aversion to cold or wind, pain in the body, stiff neck and back, rhinophonia, retching, sweat or no sweat, cough, difficult breathing, dysphoria, and tense or slow pulse. Zhang Zhongjing picked up three main symptoms from among them, saying, "The syndromes of *Taiyang* are floating pulse, painfully stiff head and neck, and aversion to cold." He then made a distinction between tense pulse and no sweat— the syndrome of febrile disease caused by cold and slow pulse and having sweat— febrile disease caused by wind, both on the *Taiyang* channel. For this reason, discarding the dross and retaining the essence is a method that cannot be overemphasized in Chinese medicine.

Eliminating the false and retaining the true: Phenomena may be misleading. True and false symptoms and signs reflected during the development of a disease are often shown simultaneously, especially when it has reached the stage of both invigorating and declining yin and yang, or when cold and heat are intermingled. Therefore, Chinese medical theories seriously warn physicians that they must discriminate between genuine and fake, discard the false and retain the true. For instance, a pseudo-heat symptom of a flushed face, hot body, dysphoria and uneasiness may appear if the preponderance of internal yin cold blocks yang outside. When a man feels hot but does not like to take off his clothes, has clean urine and discharges watery stool, with his limbs cold, an experienced physician is sure that the patient has a genuine cold belonging to the genuine-cold and pseudo-heat syndromes. He then prepares a prescription to revive yang by warmth and heat. Moreover, in case of the preponderance of internal yang heat that blocks yin outside, the patient may have an aversion to cold, chilly limbs, and constant trembling, which are symptoms of pseudo-cold. At the same time, however, he shows symptoms of a yellow tongue, thirst and short red urine, which are symptoms of genuine heat. The treatment must be to remove the heat in order to revive yin.

In the autumn of 1963, I went on business to Huarong County in central China's Hunan Province, during which time I stayed in a friend's house. His mother was already 70 years old but still could do some housework. One day, she felt full in the stomach and did not eat anything. That night, she began to shiver with cold, but she did not put on more clothes, though. She was thirsty, with her tongue dry and yellow and pulse deep, slow and forceful. My friend said that she had suffered from constipation for five days. A diagnosis showed that she had severe constipation, with internal heat running high and the preponderance of yang blocking yin, which indicated a pseudo-cold outside and genuine heat inside. Therefore, I gave a kind of decoction called *chengqitang*, a strong purgative, to the patient to improve the situation. An hour after she took the decoction, she felt an acute pain in the abdomen, but discharged a large quantity of dried feces very soon. Some time later she had one bowl of rice water and fell asleep. All the symptoms were gone the next day, and the old woman was restored five days later. As an old saying in Chinese medicine goes, excess has its emaciated image and deficiency has its excess. In other words, the actual state of affairs is sometimes mingled with false appearances. So it is necessary to discard the false and retain the true before finding the essence of a disease and making a correct diagnosis.

In addition, the transformation of contradictions in the development of a disease and the change of quality and quantity should not be neglected. As you know, a thing is a unity of two opposites, which are always in conflict with each other. As a result, one grows and the other declines, and a new thing comes into being. Nevertheless, the new thing contains the remnants of the old thing or process more or less. If we fail to see it clearly, we will not be able to discriminate between the new and the old; instead, we will take the false for the true. As often seen in medical practice, a yang disease may change into a yin one, and a yin disease into a yang one. In this process, especially when excess and deficiency change their positions in yin and yang, yin and yang syndromes exist together, and it is no easy to tell one from the other. But the experience of ancient physicians is worth studying. Take specialists in acute febrile diseases for instance. When a febrile disease enters the *qi* system, he would say that the disease is about to go into the *ying* system as long as he finds the tongue of the patient is red and purple, even though the fever is still high. Now, the decoctions *baihutang* and *chengqitang* for the clearing of heat and elimination of constipation will not work well; they must be used together with the decoctions for the clearing of the *ying* and *xue* systems and the ventilation of the *qi* system.

One point needs attention, and that is the four methods of diagnosis should be combined; otherwise, a doctor will not be able to do a good job of it, especially when he fails to observe the principles of Chinese medicine. However, the diagnosis seems one-sided sometimes because these methods are based not on modern examining means but on intuitive observation given by the doctor and the account by the patient. That is a defect in traditional Chinese medicine. Nevertheless, this can be offset more or less by careful work and rich knowledge on the part of the doctor.

Methodology in the Principles of Treatment

What we will deal with in this chapter is methodology in the principles of treatment, which are richly permeated by systematic dialectic thinking.

a) All things are related to one another, and their change depends on time, place and conditions in the principles of treatment.

Traditional Chinese medicine believes that human beings and nature are closely interrelated and that differences exist in the constitution of different human beings. Appropriate measures must be taken in treatment with regard to the difference of time, place and individual. For instance, the medicine for yang should be taken in the morning but that for yin at night. *Jimingsan* (cock-crowing power), which consists of *Semen Arecae, Pericarpium Citri Reticulatae, Fructus Chaenomelis, Fructus Evodiae, Folium Perillae, Radix Platycodi* and fresh ginger, is used to cure swelling and pain from beriberi and rheumatism. It is so called because it is usually taken at dawn when the cock crows. Why is it taken at that time? The reason is that yin becomes exhausted and yang gets alive when the cock crows. The exception is that the dosage and composition will be different from season to season. Take the wind-cold due to exogeous affection for example. The medicine should not be too pungent or warm in summer when the temperature is high and the body's muscles are loose. Under normal conditions, *Folium Perillae, Herba Schizonepetae*, fresh ginger and fermented soya beans will work. Things are different in winter when the temperature is quite low and the muscles get contracted, and only pungent and warm sudorific kinds of medicine such as *Herba Ephedrae*, *Ramulus Cinnamomi* and *Herba Asari* will serve the purpose and the dosage be large. The same is true of some other kinds of medicine. *Radix Aconiti*, *Cortex Cinnamomi*, *Herba Cistanchis* and *Herba Epimedii* cannot be taken by those suffering from the deficiency of yang in summer because they may result in an increase in the rate of death, while *Radix Rehmanniae*, *Radix Scrophulariae*, *Radix Ophiopogonis* and *Plastrum Testudinis* should not be taken by those suffering from the deficiency of yin in winter, otherwise they may have diarrhea and loss of weight.

The geographical factor should also be taken into account. Says *Huang Di Nei Jing*, "A disease should be treated with different methods. Why? The geographical factor plays a part." When giving treatment to a patient living in northwest China, a doctor should be careful about the use of cooling medicine because the climate there is quite chilly; instead, he is allowed to increase the dosage of warming and heating drugs in a proper way. If he has medical practice in the southeastern part of China where people are liable to warm-dampness syndrome due to the warm and damp climate, he should be careful about those warm and hot drugs, but when using clearing, chilling and dampness-dispelling drugs, he can increase their dosages. Originating in southeast China's Jiangsu and Zhejiang provinces, the school of acute febrile diseases has such a principle that pungent and warm drugs such as *Herba Ephedrae* and *Ramulus Cinnamomi* should be avoided for the nature of febrile diseases. Even in the same region, geological conditions are quite different from part to part; if a patient lives on the mountain where the climate is cloudy and cold and suffers from cold-dampness, he should be given pungent and warm drugs.

It should be emphatically stated that, although Chinese medical treatment pays great attention to the relationship between disease, place and time, the general principle of treatment starts from the reaction of the human body. Specific symptoms dictate the use of specific drugs.

This does not mean, however, that external symptoms caused by wind and cold, or the predominance of yin cold in summertime or on the southeastern plains cannot be treated with pungent warm diaphoretics or drugs that support yang. Nor does it imply that wind and heat symptoms or the deficiency of yin in winter in the northwestern region cannot be treated with pungent chilly diaphoretics or yin-nourishing drugs. Chinese treatment begins with the regulation of yin and yang. The use of yang and hot drugs to cure the yin syndrome and the cold syndrome, or the use of yin and cooling drugs to cure yang and heat syndromes, observes the principle of starting from the opposite to balance yin and yang. Since people are closely related to natural phenomena, the environmental influence must be taken into account when preparing prescriptions and giving drugs, and the dosage adjusted accordingly. To be a physician, "one should master the general rules and respond to the changing situation," as the medical proverb says.

When taking appropriate measures in light of the patient in question, the doctor should pay enough attention to the question on dosage. The dosage must be large for young and strong people, but small for old and weak people and children. Moreover, the location of a diseased *zang* or *fu* organ should also be a factor to be considered when deciding upon the dosage. In the mind's eyes of ancient doctors, the upper energizer is like a feature floating on the surface, the middle one like a pivot having the descent and ascent in control and the lower one like a weight where deepness and heaviness are compared, so the dosage for the lung disease should be small, the spleen or stomach disease moderate and the liver or kidney disease large. As *Huang Di Nei Jing* puts it, *qi* may run high or low, diseases exist in a near or remote place, symptoms appear inside or outside, and the dosage of medicine be small or large, and modest measures are for the upper part and drastic ones for the lower part."

However, these teachings have not attracted enough

attention from a number of doctors yet. They use a large dosage of drug for most of diseases in order to get rid of them at one stroke. Of course, if it is a serious disease, or an acute one, and the condition of the illness warrants a great effort, the dosage should appropriately be large; otherwise no good results will be gained. For ordinary or chronic diseases, however, it is not appropriate to use large dosages. If the disease is serious but the dosage of medicine is small or vice versa, the balance between yin and yang will not be achieved. In addition, some chronic diseases for which a certain *zang* or *fu* organ has been damaged for a long time should be treated step by step so that the organ can be mended. Haste does not bring success.

Some people have blind faith in tonics, thinking that they will be used to keep fit and prolong life. As a matter of fact, health depends on the balance of yin and yang and the order of *wuxing*. If tonics are given to an healthy organism, the balance between yin and yang and the original order will be disturbed; if the body is really weak, a problem still exists as to which should be tonified, yin or yang and *qi* or blood. Moreover, each kind of medicine has a dual character: positive and side effects. According to *Huang Di Nei Jing*, any medicine, if taken for a long time, may cause the accumulation of *qi*; if *qi* is accumulated for a long time, there will be much risk of death.

b) In its principle of treatment, traditional Chinese medicine is permeated by dialectic thinking. For instance, there is the law governing the reinforcement and reduction of the *zang-fu* organs, along with the one about interaction between outside and inside.

Traditional medicine maintains that all body parts are an organic whole, and their relationships are closely related, such as those between the *zang* organs, the *zang* and *fu* organs, the *fu* organs, the *zang-fu* organs and the *jingluo* system and outside and inside. These relationships include generation, inhibition, restraint and metamorphosis, and are governed by certain regularities, as well as laws of order in relationships between outside and inside. Based on these, medical methods such as the reinforcement and reduction of the *zang-fu* organs and the mutual treatment of outside and inside. In other words, when one organ is affected by a disease, the others concerned should also be given corresponding treatment.

One of the principles of reinforcement and reduction is that if deficiency is found in an organ, its "mother" organ should be reinforced; if hyperfunction found in an organ, its "child" organ should be treated with dispelling or inhibiting measures. As explained above, one element of *wuxing* is generated by the other, and the relationship between the spleen and the lung is just like that between earth and metal. If the digestion is poor, pulmonary *qi* becomes weak and there is a cough; here the method of reinforcing the spleen is to help the lung, just as earth is replenished to generate metal. One day in 1963 when I was working in Huarong County in Hunan Province, I met a 34-year-old woman who had had a cough for 18 months. I was told that many kinds of treatment had been tried in vain. The symptoms were anorexia, yellow complexion, short breath, lassitude, cough with thin whitish phlegm, light fat tongue with white coating, and tight-weak pulse. The reason for failure was that the drugs she had had were just to clear the lung, stop coughing or remove inflammation without taking the obstruction of the passage of *qi* by phlegm into account. Since pulmonary *qi* was weak, the patient could not help coughing from time to time. Then a decoction was prepared for the patient, which was made of *Radix Ginseng, Poria, Rhizoma Atractylodis Macrocephalae, Radix Glycyrrhizae, Rhizoma Pinelliae, Pericarpium Citri Reticulatae, Radix Asteris* and *Fructus Schisandrae*. After ten doses, the disease that had lingered for more than a year was cured within two weeks.

Some young people suffer from oneirogmus. This should not be attributed to a weak kidney but to hypertonic fire in the liver or heart. This is because the kidney (water) is to the liver (wood) as the mother is to the child, and dysfunction appears in *jing*-storing. If they are given astringents and hemostatics under such circumstances, no good results will be gained. A proper treatment should clear and reduce fire in the liver. If it is pacified, renal function will not be unimpeded and oneirogmus will be cured. Hepatic purgation decoction has proved effective in curing the hyperactive hepatic fire and preventing it from interfering with the seminal chamber.

Methods of mutual treatments for outside and inside are as follows: reducing outside to pacify inside, opening inside to communicate with outside and clearing inside to relieve outside. These are based on the fact that outside and inside are counterparts; methods are thus adopted to treat the *fu* organs when the disease affects the *zang* organs, the *zang* organs when it affects the *fu* organs. Take the lung and the large intestine for instance. They are related to each other as outside to inside. If heat is accumulated in the large intestine and the feces becomes dry and constipated, *qi* of the lung will be obstructed and cough appears. If treatment begins with the lung, good results will hardly be achieved. Generally, drugs such as *lianggesan* (diaphragm-cooling power) are given to reduce the heat in the large intestine, which may help get pulmonary *qi* to flow and cure cough.

Constipation can be caused by congested *qi* in the lung and will not be effectively cured by merely treating the large intestine. Instead, prescriptions that open up inside (lung) and gain access to outside (large intestine) are better. Sun Simiao has this to say about a simple prescription in *Qian Jin Yao Fang*: "If a woman suffers from difficult urination, she can take a kind of power made up of *Radix Asteris* diluted with well water. That has proved quite effective." *Radix Asteris* can be used to check the upward surge of *qi* along the Lung Channel of Hand-*Taiyin*, and remove the urinary obstruction, because the lung belongs to the upper stream of body fluid, and when pulmonary *qi* is elevated, water will flow up naturally.

Some treating methods sound incredible in Chinese medicine. Eye diseases are cured by treating the liver and kidney, ear diseases by treating the kidney, nose diseases by treating the lung and diseases in the mouth and on the tongue by treating the heart and spleen, among other things. Toothache due to the deficiency of the kidney and the flare-up of internal fire and gingival abscess due to the steam from gastric fire, for example, can be treated with cold drugs and renal tonifiers. These are also regarded as instances of outside-inside mutual treatment.

Ample attention should be paid to the other principle that the lower part of the body is treated when the disease appears in the upper part, and vice versa. For example, when *qi* and fire flow up and bring blood with them, massive hemorrhage takes place in the upper digestive and respiratory tracts such as hematemesis, hemoptysis and nosebleeding. To treat this disease, purgative drugs like rhubarb should be given to depress the *qi* and fire; fresh rhubarb has proved its worth in treating hemorhage. The reason is that rhubarb acting on the locus of the colon causes hyperemia in the lower part and therefore reduces blood circulation in the upper part so as to make hemostasis possible. Asthma as mentioned above can be cured by tonifying the kidney to improve inspiration. Another case in point is proctoptosis due to the sinking of the spleen *qi* which is usually treated by tonifying the spleen and replenishing *qi* to elevate the spleen *qi*.

c) Traditional treatment is permeated with recognition of the unity of opposites, mutual conditioning and alternation of contradictions. Chinese medicine believes that diseases are the struggle between two antagonistic opposites: body resistance and pathogenic factors. If body resistance exists, pathogenic factors retreat; if pathogenic factors prevail, resistance becomes weak. *Huang Di Nei Jing* says: "Excess syndromes occur when pathogenic factors are in abundance, but deficiency syndromes take place when the patient's *jing* and *qi* are severely damaged." Therefore, the principle of inhancing the body resistance to get rid of pathogenic factors is used in Chinese medicine. Inhancing resistance means the use of medication, nutriment, acupuncture and moxibustion, *qigong*, massage and physical training to improve the constitution, elevate the body's ability to adapt to the external and internal environment and keep fit. That is why this principle can be adopted for symptoms showing feeble resistance. Old and weak people are liable to cold, and they may come down with it even when they fail to tuck themselves in bed at night or are slow to get dressed in the morning. If the doctor tries to dispel wind-cold without taking into account tonificaton, he cannot help the patient get rid of pathogenic factors once for all, even though his methods are correct. This is simply because the resistance within the body is too weak to get pathogenic factors out of it. In fact, the decoction *yupingfengtang* made up of *Radix Astragali, Rhizoma Atractylodis Macrocephalae* and *Radix Ledebouriellae* is of much help to him if it is taken for a long time.

Getting rid of pathogenic factors means the dispelling of pathogens and the restoring of resistance. That includes such methods as diaphoresis, purgation, induced vomiting, purification, and digestion and dredging. If a patient is not abstemious in eating or drinking and has a poor digestion, he will feel full in the stomach and chest with fever, sweating and even loss of consciousness. That is an excess syndrom of the stomach. Now he cannot be treated through tonification but given the decoction *chengqitang* instead, which helps reduce pathogenic factors and improve health.

Improving resistance and dispelling pathogenic factors is an organic whole and should be used together. Generally speaking, both of them should be taken into account in medical treatment and preferance given to one over the other. Nevertheless, we can find something quite different in the history of Chinese medicine. Some doctors laid emphasis on the enhancement of resistance such as Li Gao (1190-1251) and Zhang Jingyue of the school of reinforcement and Zhu Danxi (1282-1358) of the school of yin nourishment. Others attached importance to removing pathogenic factors such as Zhang Zihe (1156-1228) who was famous for his diaphoretic, emetic and purgation therapies. Some doctors in ancient China paid much attention to one of the two methods and had their own styles of treatment, but this does not mean they viewed the other with disdain.

Body resistance and pathogenic factors, and deficiency and excess have something to do with each other. Weak resistance may lead to deficiency, and too many pathogenic factors may weaken resistance and result in deficiency. Both the enhancement of resistance and the dispelling of pathogenic factors should be taken into consideration when treating the deficiency syndromes. If resistance is too weak to get rid of pathogenic factors, the enhancement of resistance should be emphasized when treating the excess syndromes by dispelling pathogenic factors. If resistance is too weak and pathogenic factors are too many, a doctor should take the occasion to deal with the situation, for to dispell pathogenic factors may lead to a smore serious deficiency but to improve resistance may result in the existance of pathogenic factors. When a patient suffering from pneumonia is in a state of shock with pathogenic factors in abundance, there is a danger of sudden collapse of resistance. A decoction like single ginseng should be given to keep the patient alive while awaiting further treatment. Only when he has recovered from shock can measures be taken against the pathogenic factors. According to Chinese medical theories, inhancing resistance and dispelling pathogenic factors can be done at the same time or one after the other, all depending on concrete conditions. A general principle is that no pathogenic factors should be retained when improving resistance and no harm done to resistance when getting rid of the factors.

Let us now consider the principle of treating yin and yang in terms of their unity in opposition.

With invasion of pathogenic factors, human yin and yang are damaged with one excessive and the other deficient, and then diseases appear. A principle is to regulate the relationship between yin and yang and create balance between them. There are quite a few symptoms when yin and yang lose balance, but the most important are that the preponderance of yin gives rise to a cold syndrome but that of yang causes a heat syndrome, and the deficiency of yin brings on internal heat but that of yang causes external cold. That is to say that a heat or cold syndrome will appear when yin or yang gets ill. Specifically, the preponderance of yang may damage yin fluids, as shown in a patient of high fever with dry and red tongue and dry and yellow fur. Better results will be gained when yin-nourishing herbal drugs like *Radix Rehmanniae, Radix Ophiopogonis, Radix Scrophulariae* and *Radix Glehniae* are added to those for eliminating toxic heat. On the other hand, the deficiency of yin may lead to the hyperfunction of yang, and general symptoms are consumptive fever, night sweat, red cheeks, cough, spitting blood, dysphoria, fever, hunger, pain and heat in the foot and knee, red tongue, and rapid and forceful pulse at the *chi* position. Such a case is often treated with a large dose of yin-nourishing pills, which consists of *Rhizoma Anemarrhenae, Cortex Phellodendri, Radix Rehmanniae, Plastrum Testudinis* and pig spine marrow with honey. In this prescription, *Rhizoma Anemarrhenae* and *Cortex Phellodendri* are antipyretics for the reduction of heat and protection of yin, while *Radix Rehmanniae* and *Plastrum Testudinis* are for the nourishment of yin and harmony of yang.

The damage of yang due to the exuberance of yin and the deficiency of yang has quite a few symptoms such as limbs in syncope, aversion to cold, sleeping with the body huddled, retching and vomiting, watery diarrhea, deep but faint pulse. Decoctions like *sinitang* of *Radix Aconiti, Radix Glycyrrhizae* and *Rhizoma Zingiberis* are used to prevent yang from collapsing. For another instance, a patient suffering from the deficiency of yang of the kidney usually has diarrhea before dawn because he can hardly bear yin cold. The drugs for warm and hot pathogenic factors like the pill *sishenwan* are often used to treat the disease, which contains *Fructus Psoraleae, Fructus Evodiae, Semen Myristicae, Fructus Schisandrae*, ginger and *Fructus Zizyphi Jujubae*. That is to treat cold with heat and dispel yin in excess by warming yang.

According to the Chinese medical theory, yin and yang depend on each other for generation, and without yang there is no yin and vice versa. Health is good when yin is even and well and yang firm; life ceases when yin and yang are separate. The relationship between yin and yang is quite important in medical treatment. In addition, the kidney is the foundation of the inborn constitution. The yin of the other organs depends on renal yin for nourishment and their yang on renal yang for warmth. That is why renal yin and yang are also called genuine yin and yang and play a key role in the function of yin and yang in the body. This requires people to take renal yin into account when they warm and reinforce renal yang. A pill called *jinkuishenqiwan* from *Jin Kui Yao Lue Fang Lun*, for one, is often used to cure beriberi, retention of phlegm and fluid, diabetes, thirst, fetal rotation and weak pulse at the *chi* position in addition to lumbago, flaccity and cold in the lower limbs, cramp in the lower abdomen, and difficulty in urination. This pill, made up of *Radix Aconiti Praeparata* and *Cortex Cinnamomi* is to reinforce renal yang, along with *Radix Rehmanniae* and *Fructus Corni* for the nourishment of renal yin. Another example is epidemic fever whose pathogenic factors, if existing for a long time, may scorch real yin and cause wind symptoms due to the deficiency of blood. As a result, spasm appears, hands and feet wriggle, and the tongue become purple. A general method is to prescribe the decoction *dadingfengzhutang*, which consists of *Radix Rehmanniae, Radix Ophiopogonis, Radix Paeoniae Alba, Colla Corii Asini*, egg, *Plastrum Testudinis* and *Carapax Trionycis* to nourish yin and supplement blood, and *Concha Ostreae, Fructus Schisandrae* and *Plastrum Testudinis* to check the exuberance of yang. In case of the flare-up of fire due to the deficiency of yin which may cause hectic fever, bone steaming, withered waist and weak knees, dizziness and dazed eyes, chattering teeth and dry pharynx, a decoction consisting of *Radix Anemarrhenae, Cortex Phellodendri* and *Radix Rehmanniae* is usually used to nourish yin and reduce the fire. If the fire abates, however, cooling drugs like *Radix Anemarrhenae* and *Phellodendri* should be laid aside so as to prevent too much fire from impairing renal yang and make both renal yin and yang deficient. There are two types of fire in Chinese medicine: deficient and excessive. The fire of excess type means that there is too much yang, so bitter cold drugs like *Rhizoma Coptidis, Radix Scutellariae* and *Cortex Phellodendri* are used to reduce yang heat; that of deficiency type does not refer to the abundance of yang but the deficiency of yin fluid, and the nourishment yin can restore the balance between yin and yang, and the disease is cured.

Another kind of disease is caused by the disharmony between yin and yang, a problem which involves the composition of the yin and yang systems but cannot be solved simply through reinforcement and reduction. There is a patient suspected of suffering from neurosis feels cold one moment and has a fever the other, with the pulse tight. Now the mediation method may be more effective than others, and according to this principle, powders called *sinisan* and *xiaoyaosan* are prescribed to the patient and good results are gained.

d) A universal principle in traditional Chinese medicine is to find out the key element that affects health in treatment. It is in conformity with the theory that there is one aspect of key importance in a thing, and one thing or process of this kind among many.

(1) An illness may have several symptoms and signs. If we start to cure a disease when we just see its symptoms— by curing the head when the head aches and the

foot when the foot aches— we will not be able to get rid of it. Chinese physicians are taught not only to discover the symptoms of a disease, but to learn about the relationship between them and the essence of the disease before giving correct treatment.

(2) A disease may have more than one symptom and a patient may have a number of diseases at the same time. However, only one of them plays a key role in the development of a disease or the recovery from the illness. That is what is implied in the principle that the main element effecting health should be found in treatment.

(3) Different diseases may have almost the same symptoms in different patients, showing that there are basically common reactions in the body. This tells that we can adopt almost the same methods to treat them. Of course, some differences exist in the symptoms, and the dosage should be different in the light of actual conditions.

(4) A single disease may have different syndromes in different patients. This is chiefly because there are differences between the patients in constitution and body reaction. In addition, different syndromes may also appear in the different stages of a desease because of different reactions from the organism. As the cause is different, they cannot be treated identically.

The recent trend of medical development in China is towards the combination of Chinese and Western medicine. In accordance with the principle of different kinds of treatment for identical diseases, several main prescriptions for the same diseases have been worked out. This provides convenience for both doctors and patients, and also marks an improvement over the past practice of treating the same disease with one or two kinds of medicine to the neglect of the difference of constitution and syndrome. In spite of this, a doctor should first master Chinese medical theories, principles, prescriptions and medicine so that they can avoid blindness in practice and make correct diagnosis of a diesease. There are also many set prescriptions and ready-made drugs in Chinese medicine, which were often used by ancient doctors, but with the ingredients and dosage changed in light of actual conditions. Xu Lingtai (1693-1771), a well-known doctor living in the Qing Dynasty said on one occasion, "It is necessary to know whether the symptoms of your patient are completely the same as those described in ancient prescriptions. If so, you can use the set prescriptions; otherwise you will make adjustment or write new ones." That each disease has different symptoms and each patient has several diseases should also be taken into account when you use set prescriptions. Moreover, there are such cases that principles are the same but prescriptions are different, and prescriptions are the same but dosages are different. All these should be kept in mind.

(5) Attention should be also paid to the relationship between the incidental and the fundamental on the one hand and the urgent and the less urgent on the other. The fundamental refers to the root cause of a disease, the old disease, the internal organs and body resistance, and to learn about the fundamental aspect of a disease or the main one among many diseases may help get rid of the disease(s), while the incidental means the symptoms and signs of the disease, the new disease, the body surface and pathogenic factors. Treating a disease in light of the fundamental helps recover once for all, but doing the same thing in light of the incidental only gives temporary relief. As for the urgent and the less urgent, their relationship is dialectic: treat acute symptoms first in emergency cases, but deal with its fundamental cause when they are relieved. This is because everything in a disease is always in motion, and treating methods should be given in accordance with the situation. A doctor should find out the root cause of a disease when it develops quite slowly. Take asthenia with internal injury for instance. Its symptoms are the deficiency of yin, high fever and cough, and the development is quite slow. The fever and cough belong to the incidental but the deficiency of yin to the fun-

damental. Just paying attention to cough without taking into account the deficiency of yin will make complete cure impossible.

Treating acute symptoms first in emergency cases can only be used when the less important becomes the important all of a sudden. It may be temperory yet should be dealt with at once because it develops too fast to admit of delay. That is why acute symptoms should be alleviated first at the critical moment. If a patient suffering from hepatitis suddenly finds himself in a state of ascites with short breath, constipation, and dysuria, he should be treated for ascites, though it is only one symptom of hepatic. The reason is that the respiratory, digestive, circulatory and urinary systems as well as water electrolyte metabolism will be disturbed and life itself endangered. Now ascites is the key to the question, and everything should be done to make it less grievous before concentrating on hepatitis. Taken as a whole, ascites is secondary to hepatitis, and it will be of frequent recurrence unless the main disease is cured. So attention should be given to the protection of the liver when treating ascites.

Of course, there is such a situation that both the fundamental and the incidental are acute, and it is impossible to take care of one to the neglect of the other. Take a nephritic patient for example. If he is afflicted with wind-cold when his nephritis is still quite grievous, the symptoms will be aversion to cold, cough, fullness in the chest, lumbago, oliguria and anarsaca. According to Chinese medical theory, renal edema is fundamental but obstruction by wind-cold is incidental, and yet, treating either of them can hardly solve the problem. This requires a doctor to have them treated at the same time, with the pathogenic factors dispelled from the exterior of the body to ventilate the lung on the one hand and yang warmed to dissolve the water on the other. There are times when the disease is not urgent, and the doctor may take both the fundamental and the incidental into account at the same time in treatment. Take low fever due to the deficiency of yin for instance. The deficiency of yin is fundamental and low fever is incidental. You can allay fever by nourishing yin, but that will take a long time. A better method is to have antipyretics along with yin-nourishing drugs.

There are some differences between treating acute symptoms first in emergency and then its fundamental cause when they are relieved on the one hand and treating both incidental and fundamental aspects on the other. However, their point is the same and that is to solve the main problem in light of the development of a disease, and at the same time lay groundwork for the tackling of the other ones.

Chapter V

THE SCIENTIFIC SIGNIFICANCE OF TRADITIONAL METHODOLOGY

We have discussed the methods of traditional Chinese medicine. It is clear that the yin-yang theory plays an important role in the establishment of the Chinese medical theoretical system based on unity of opposites and the order of systems and has therefore become the heart of the system. The *zangxiang* theory is about physiology and pathology, which was formed after the relationships between the human body and nature and body surface and internal organs, and the functional connections between generation, inhibition, restraint and dissolution became known from outside to inside and from one to the other. The *bianzhenglunzhi* theory, which has those on yin and yang and *zangxiang* as its basis, is quite unique in the understanding of syndrome and causes, diagnosis and treatment. In the past, there were controversies in Chinese medical circles as to which is the theoretical kernel of traditional Chinese medicine. Some said it was the *zangxiang* theory; others believed that it was the yin-yang theory; and still others, the *bianzhenglunzhi* theory. I am of the opinion that these three theories are inseparable. The yin-yang theory is the basis of traditional methodology; the *zangxiang* theory is the basis of its physiology and pathology; and the *bianzhenglunzhi* theory is its therapeutic basis. The three theories, interrelated and interdependent, serve as part and parcel of the Chinese medical theoretical system. In fact, what the system includes are many more than those— prescriptions, Chinese pharmacology, internal medicine, surgery, gynacology, pediatrics, acupuncture, moxibustion, massage, medico-athletics and health maintenance, but they are all guided by the three basic theories which have been dealt with in the above chapters.

Traditional Chinese medicine has been regarded as an empirical medical science, something that can be explained in various ways. That Western medicine is called experimental medicine as it is based on experiment, while traditional Chinese medicine is seen as empirical medicine because it is formed on the basis of practical experience, but the point of view that Chinese medicine is just a medical technology based on perceptual knowledge without a theoretical system is not acceptable. This question is simple to clarify as long as we have a brief review of the history of both Chinese and Western medicine.

Ancient Western medicine may date back to the period between the sixth and fourth centuries B.C., when the Hippocratic School of Greece advocated the theory of the four natural elements— earth, water, wind and fire, which were said to form four properties— dryness, dampness, cold and warmth. These four properties were believed to form the four humors in human body -- melancholy or black bile, choler or yellow bile, phlegm, and blood. Hippocrates believed that if the components and forces of these four elements, properties and fluids were harmonious, people would be in good health; otherwise, they would fall ill. During the Alexandria Period (3rd-1st century B.C.), many people began to study anatomy, and one of the schools was named after Erasistratus, who adopted an ancient theory about essence and vitality. Later, at the Christian Era, the Roman school of Galen tried to apply anatomy and physiology to medical practice in order to make the then medical theory rational. However, Galen had the theory of four elements and that of essence and vitality as the basis of its physiological theory. After the fall of the Roman Empire in the West in 476, history entered the Dark Ages, which lasted about 1,000 years; during the Middle Ages, medicine was the servant of religion and received little development. After the Renaissance, anatomy, physiology and some other sciences had some development, but it was not until the 19th century that researchers spent too much time on theory and their points of view changed from time to time. As a result, no basic theoretical system had ever appeared that could be accepted by most of doctors, so experience was something to go by in clinical diagnosis, and doctors had to work according to the principle of Hippocrates so as to help improve man's natural ability to regain health early in the 19th century. It was after the 19th century that the theoretical system of modern medicine began to take shape, along with the development of modern science.

Chinese medicine is quite different. Its theoretical system has never changed greatly since it was formed in *Huang Di Nei Jing* during the Qin and Han period though there was unrest in those years, and yin and yang, *zangxiang* and *bianzhenglunzhi* have been the basis of various schools of medicine in China.

The difference of development between Western and Chinese medicine can be found in the history of culture and idea. Ancient Greece's naive dialectics and materialism, due to their inherent defects, were replaced by idealism and metaphysics. The naive materialistic dialectic thought of traditional Chinese medicine has likewise undergone a history of two or three thousand years, during which there was a long period of feudalism and semi-feudalism and semi-colony. It also drew an attack from various kinds of idealism and metaphysics, and was even banned by the government, but it survived, though its development was quite slow. All this would be difficult to understand if the peculiars of the theoretical system and the therapeutic effects of traditional Chinese medicine are overlooked.

Why is it that Greek philosophy and traditional Chinese medicine met such different fates? Isn't the dialectical thinking of Chinese medicine also naive? Isn't it devoid of modern scientific argumentation in many details, just like Greek philosophy was? Isn't it groundless in some ways? The key to all these questions lies in the fact that traditional Chinese medicine has never ceased serving the broad masses since it appeared. Therapeutic practice concerns the life and death of people, so no exaggeration or unrealisticness whatsoever is permissible. Knowledge comes from practice, and the theoretical system and treating methods of traditional Chinese medicine become rich in practice with the help of doctors and experts of various periods. Traditional Chinese medicine originates from naive dialectics but, with the development of society, has surpassed it. Therefore this medicine has its own style of treatment: observing in an intuitive way but thinking in a scientific one, and viewing the disease as a whole but analyzing concretely. We can say that all this is the treasure of the Chinese civilization. There is every need to develop its traditional medicine so that it will better serve the health of mankind.

Armed with modern science and technology, such as the electronic microscope and physics, chemistry and mathematics in experiments, research in Western medicine has now become increasingly deep— from the cellular level to subcellular and molecular ones and there are more and more branches of science, with the structure and change of basic substances like molecules and electric currents learned about at the context of microworld. This marks a new and significant stage of development. Everything, however, has its opposite. With the classification of medicine becoming more detailed and research more varified, we are liable to see the trees but the not forest unless dialectic materialism is the guiding principle of our work. That is to spend much time on those we are studying but neglect the relationship between the organism's various aspects.

Engels pointed out in his book *Dialektik und Natur*, "The ejection of seeds— the embryo and the animal produced by birth are not to be conceived as a 'part' that is separated from the 'whole,' which would give a distorted treatment. It becomes a part only in a dead body." He said that a chemist can dissolve a slice of flesh before concluding that flesh is made from oxygen, carbon, hydrogen, nitrogen, etc. Yet these elements, if separated, would not be flesh any more. He further stated that life is the highest form of the motion of matter, and in it are included lower forms of motion such as mechanics, physics and chemistry, though life should not be reduced to these forms. Modern systematics holds that the nature and law of a thing as a whole depend only on the interrelation and interaction of its various factors, which are not reflected in the sum total of the properties and activities of its component parts. Scientific methodology tells us that the deeper research goes, the more important the internal relations of a thing are. This has been verified in the development of modern science and technology.

The development of science during the period between the Renaissance and the early years of the 20th century was the expansion of science and technology and the deepening of research in various disciplines, but that over the 50 years changed a lot with science getting synthesized and transectional. Modern science and technology are characterized by mutual infiltration and inseparableness. Quite a few marginal disciplines have appeared, reflecting a tendency towards ramification that is in turn an expressing form of synthesization. The integration of ramification and synthesization pushes science to a more highly unified system, and all disciplines have common language, concepts and methods. All these lead to the systematization of modern science. Modern scientists, for example, have discovered four fundamental forces of interaction among particles that are known: gravitational, electromagnetic, and the strong and weak forces that bond components of nuclei. This discovery requires scientists to explore the possibility of unified field that explains the four forces.

These trends make it necessary to establish new scientific methods on the basis of traditional ones. That requires scientists to follow the law of "negation of negation," surpassing metaphysics to once more accept materialist dialectics as a guide. Since the 1930s and 1940s, the appearance of transectional sciences like cybernetics, informatics and systematics reflected the need for new methodology, and these sciences demonstrated the existence of more internal relations and laws of motion in nature, regarding the object of study as a complete, organic and complex system. In so doing, they find methods of solving problems in communication and control systems, and introduced quantitative analysis into some branches of science. That is a leap forward in methodology.

This development is also reflected in modern medicine. There is horizontal research in Western medicine, but its emphasis is on the study of the human body in a longitudinal way. In other words, every body is divided into systems and every system dissected into organs, tissues and cells. All this makes progress possible in all fields of Western medicine. In addition, following the development of medical science, the classification of diseases is becoming increasingly narrow. With this, a doctor may get a better understanding of various organs and tissues as well as diseases but one-sidedness is unavoidable. That means lacking a general understanding of the relationships between man and nature, various systems, and between diseases. Depth and scope are two aspects of equal importance in scientific development. If we pay attention to the depth of knowledge but neglect its scope, results are not satisfactory. For example, much time is spent on the relations between pathogenic microorganisms and some body part but little time on their relations with nature which has a constant effect on the body and microorganisms; much time is spent on different human organs but little time on the acquisition of man's whole image made up of the relations between the organs; much time is spent on the histopathological features of each disease but little time on the study of the "patient" who lives in this world and has complicated mental activities.

All these are detrimental to the development of medical science and the enhancement of treatment.

Attention is paid to the study of the system as a whole but not to that of the body in a longitudinal way. As a result, it is easy to have it linked and integrated with cybernetics, informatics, systematics and other modern sciences. Recently, some scientists show great enthusiasm for Chinese medical theories, calling the *wuxing* theory a naive ordinary systematics. Others, who have studied the *jingluo* theory for quite a long time from the viewpoint of informatics, believe that the *jingluo* system serves as the body's control system with *qi* and blood similar to "information" and its carriers, with channels and collaterals to information channels and acupoints to the input and output.

There are still some naive dialectical elements in Chinese medical theories now. But we have no reason to feel sorry for their slow progress; instead, we should know that the theories and methods employed in Chinese medicine are important in scientific research. For our purpose is not to be sentimental over China's past or traditional medicine but to summarize the experience and lessons acquired from the history of science. In the rapid development of modern medicine there is still a need of studying traditional theories and methods.

All specific problems in traditional Chinese medicine have yet to be expounded by the theories and technology of modern science. Take the liver for instance. According to the *zangxiang* theory, it has a specific body opening in the eyes and stores the soul, with its condition determining that of the tendons and outward manifestation reflected in the nails. Their internal relations have proved their existence in practice, but their quality awaits careful study; when we make a further study of them, we will know both the hows and whys.

Chapter VI

SIGNIFICANCE OF THEORY AND METHOD IN CHINESE MEDICINE

Presentation of the Problem

Here we will explore the road of development and direction of reform in traditional Chinese medicine in terms of theories and methods and fundamental substance and regularities, in order to draw attention from the medical community and provoke discussion.

Since 1949, the Chinese government has paid attention to traditional Chinese medicine and pharmacology, pointing out that they are a great national treasure and that efforts should be made to explore their contents and improve their quality. At the same time, the Chinese government has put forward a suggestion that Chinese and Western medicine be combined to establish a new medicine and pharmacology.

Since the 1950s, there have appeared quite a few hospitals and institutes specialized in traditional medicine in China. Together with them, many teachers and researchers have been organized to work, students trained, classical medical books published, teaching materials compiled for use in medical institutes and veteran Chinese medical doctors called to sum up their experience. All this promotes scientific research in traditional Chinese medicine, especially in the *jingluo* system, acupuncture and moxibustion, *zang-fu* organs, the method of promoting blood flow to eliminate blood stasis, the treatment of bone fractures with small splints.

However, there are problems in the development of Chinese medicine. Manfred Porkert, Professor of Sinology and Chinese Medical Theory at Munich University, visited China in 1978. After his return, he spoke of the following problem with great concern: I was particularly impressed by the patient and sincere modesty of Chinese doctors qualified in Western medicine, and now studying or exercising Chinese medicine, by the devotion to the cause of the medical tradition of all the personnel working in institutions dealing with traditional medicine. This made me feel all the more painfully the striking and all-pervading imbalance in the People's Rebpulic between Western and Chinese medicine— an imbalance manifestly belying the November 1958 directive of the Central Committee, belying even more Mao Zedong's tenet that Chinese medicine must be considered a "treasury" of inherited knowledge. In fact, the November 1958 directive of the Central Committee urged that traditional Chinese and Western medicine should be applied, taught and investigated on equal terms throughout the country. This directive was preceded by a few years of a startling renaissance of the ancient tradition, which since then, in spite of apparent compliance with Party directives, is withering from within.

For various reasons, such unsettling problems as "the lack of study of the art of traditional Chinese medicine" and "the lack of trained traditional Chinese physicians" spread throughout the country. We cannot help asking how traditional Chinese medicine withstood the attempts to ban it. With its theoretical and technical powers it continued to exist and develop further. Why is it that after the new Chinese government extended so much care and support to the development of traditional medical enterprises and inaugurated so many higher schools and research institutes, traditional Chinese medical personnel dropped from 500,000 in the early 1950's to around 300,000 two or three years ago? Shouldn't we search for the cause and find the answer to this serious question?

Perhaps it is because old Chinese medicine was not scientific from the very beginning, and that due to its own defects, it was doomed to be inferior to the developed scientific Western medicine and therefore hopelessly on the decline. Traditional theories were drawn from practical experience and subsequently formed into a unique system. Because these experiences have all been tested on actual patients, it is incorrect to say that traditional medicine has not been built on scientific grounds.

How do we explain the troubling statement that "the development of the art of traditional Chinese medicine has come to an end" and that "there are no new students trained as traditional Chinese physicians?" What is the future trend of traditional medicine? These questions should be considered from a theoretical and methodological point of view instead of a technological one only; otherwise Chinese medical science can hardly gain solid development.

Characteristics of Chinese Medicine and Its Trend

In a preface to his book, Prof. Qian Xuesen says that the theoretical system of traditional Chinese medicine cannot be seen as a science in the modern sense though it has lots of scientific elements. It is instead a classical philosophy of nature, and should continue to exist because no other theory can take its place. That is why traditional Chinese medicine has to be modernized yet.

What does he mean by saying so? "Philosophy of nature" refers to the theory of a natural system. It developed during a period between the 17th century and the early years of the 19th century and was inseparable from philosophy and many fields of natural science from the very beginning. However, natural science was then underdeveloped and unable to explain many phenomena and processes and their relations in a scientific way. Therefore, philosophers and scientists attempted to use the scientific information they had acquired and philosophical speculations to explain the system of nature. When natural science did not fully develop and many things in nature remained unknown, the imaginary relations behind the phenomena and processes were not clear for the real ones in natural philosophy. This is quite understandable. For that matter, these natural philosophers predicted many scientific inventions and discoveries which were later developed. Of course, there were many mistakes because science and culture were undeveloped then. As science progressed, people began to realize that science could help them explain the system of nature satisfactorily. For example, they might explain the world as a whole and guide the system perfectly by means of dialectical materialism. Natural philosophy then became obsolete and went out of existence gradually.

Traditional Chinese medicine contains a huge system of theories, but some of them have not been explained from a scientific point of view. Its theoretical system was also built on the imaginary relations behind the body and between nature and mankind and the observation of relations that really exist as well as doctors' experience. This shows that traditional medicine has something characteristic of natural science in a sense.

Much of the theoretical system of traditional Chinese medicine has analogy and inference as its basic methods. A doctor's observation and evaluation comes from his application of *bianzhenglunzhi* theory, cognition of "syndromes" and experience as well as reaction from the organism. In fact, even if the diagnosis and principles of treatment by different doctors are basically identical for an identical patient, there might be much difference in the composition and administration of prescriptions, which will be reflected in the therapeutic effect. Some compare Western medicine to modernized industrial production, which uses standardized operations and the same products, while traditional Chinese medicine is often compared to a handicraft with more artistic characteristics. That is one of characteristic features of natural philosophy of traditionzal Chinese medicine.

Some people think otherwise, believing that natural philosophy will be replaced by modern natural science and Chinese medicine by Western medicine. They even say that only when Chinese medicine becomes systematized with the help of Western medical theories and methods can it be saved from disappearing, and that is the so-called combination of of Chinese and Western medicine.

This point of view has a methodological origin. Modern science has dissection and analysis as its basic methods, which have helped clarify the internal structure and quality of different organs, and, at this point, got the better of natural philosophy.

Qian Xuesen wrote in an article: "We have seen progress in biology. The methods of reductionism and empiricism, or themethodsof metaphysics, as R. Rosen pointed out, occupied the premdominant position in the research of natural sciences since the 18th century. That was very progressive at the time…. By the 1940's and 1950's, dissection had been used with the analysis of the layer of molecules. We can say now that we have acquired great achievements and a new science called molecular biology has appeared. The more rich our knowledge of a thing, the farther we are away from it as a whole in our research. That was realized by Bertalanffy 50 years ago. He began to study the so-called 'theoretische biologic' in 1932, regarding a living thing and its environment as a great system. He therefore created a science of general system theory, with which to probe into important questions such as human physiology, human psychology and social phenomena."

The above passage presents a clear outline of the development of science. Reductionism as a predominating method has contributed to the development of modern science, but it has its own shortcomings. Albert Szent-

Györgyi also realized this, saying, "There are large holes in our basic knowledge. It is possible that there are defects in our entire view of life. In the past, we were probably 'fishing outside of the net.' In the drama of life, a biomacromolecule is more like a stage rather than a player." (cf. *Electrobiology and Cancer*) This being the case, scientific progress demands the use of materialist dialectics and the method of systematics to free itself from this predicament. Cybernetics, informatics and systematics, which have developed rapidly since the 1930s and 1940s, repudiate the formerly used methods of analysis and reduction. Such methods are used to analyse things by combining them into a general system of interrelations and actions, and then by recognizing that the system itself actually exists and develops in an interwoven labyrinth of multiple layers and factors. Methods of general system theory may be summed up as follows: a) principle of totality, b) principle of interrelations, c) principle of order, and d) principle of the dynamic state. All these principles should be widely used in research.

General system theory, developed from the foundation of biological research, associates the order and technology of biology and the phenomena of life with the stability of the structure of the system, and is directly related to cybernetics and informatics. Systematics has now become important in the research of the phenomena of life and medicine. However, by force of habit, systematics has not yet been widely adopted in ordinary medical practice or research and included in medical textbooks. Many researchers have discovered that cybernetics, informatics and systematics are used in traditional Chinese medicine, which may help explain why it has existed over a thousand years and are receiving due attention from many scientists in the world. In short, methodology is important in traditional Chinese medicine, and a review of the history of its development will help solve other problems.

People had realized by the end of the 19th century that traditional Chinese medicine and pharmacology were great treasures. At the same time, they had kept abreast with the developments in Western medicine and tried to merge the two. For instance, Tang Zonghai (1847-1897), a well-known doctor in the Qing Dynasty, tried to substantiate the theories recorded in *Huang Di Nei Jing* by means of dissection and physiology in his book *Zhong Xi Yi Hui Tong Yi Jing Jing Yi* ("Essentials of Confluent Traditional Chinese and Western Medicine"). Another example was Zhu Peiwen (1805-?), a doctor of the Qing Dynasty, combined Western anatomy with the study of *zangxiang* in Chinese medicine in his book *Hua Yang Zang Fu Tu Xiang Yue Zuan* ("A Brief Account of the Chinese and Western Anatomy"). Their motive was good but the effect was not so. They made absurd mistakes because they did not know that Chinese and Western medicine are completely different in medical system. This problem was clarified with the theory of cybernetics in Chinese medicine. According to some experts, the method employed in Chinese medicine is mainly to study and control without opening the black box, while the one in Western medicine is to open the black box to observe the body's physiology and pathology. If we do not recognize this difference or know the reasoning behind the *zangxiang* or tell *zangxiang* from anatomy, we will make many mistakes.

Much attention has been paid to the study of traditional Chinese medicine and the combination of Chinese and Western medicine since 1949. Both the government at various levels and social organizations offered much help in many ways, which plays a big role in the development of Chinese medicine. But this does not mean that there are not any problems at all; instead, some problems are quite serious. One of them is lack of trained and competent doctors.

More recently, Professor Zhang Xiangtong, a well-known cranial physiologist, made use of electrophysiological and biochemical methods to study acupuncture analgesia. He discovered that when the relevant acupoint is pierced, the hypothalamus can be stimulated to secrete a substance which numbs the nerves and makes the correlated locus insensitive to pain. This shows that the action of acupuncture analgesia is indirect; it takes the cerebrum for the center. The body's holistic function thus moves beyond regional tissues.

It is obvious that different theoretical systems have different methods. If the methods of Western medicine are applied to the theories of traditional Chinese medicine without taking the difference between the two, half the results will be gained with twice the efffort.

As Chinese pharmacology started rather early, we can hardly recognize the pharmacodynamics and function of Chinese herbal drugs by means of modern science and technology which are mainly used to analyze and reduce the components, chemical structure and properties of Chinese drugs as well as the effects produced by those components on internal organs, tissues and cells of human body. This is chiefly because modern methods are suitable for the analysis of individual drugs and Chinese doctors' knowledge of drugs comes from experience. It is based on the action of the different drugs in adjusting the relations between yin and yang, deficiency and excess, outside and inside, cold and heat, ascent and descent, and opening and closing that Chinese doctors discovered *siqi* and *wuwei* of drugs. On the other hand, their knowledge about pharmacodynamics cannot be acquired when the body's or medicine's black box is opened, either. In fact, drugs are used as a kind of input information, and feedback is acquired with the help of Chinese medical theories and methods. Secondly, treatment is usually based on single-taste drugs in Western medicine. That is quite different from Chinese medicine in which drugs are often prescribed by reference to the syndrome, cause, site and pathology of the disease. Prescriptions are compounded on the basis of the harmonization of *jun, chen, zuo* and *shi*, and *qiqing*. A prescription is usually made up of drugs with different tastes, which, related to one another and mutually conditioning, are combined to cure the disease. In addition, Chinese drugs are mostly composed of plants and animals which themselves have several components. To analyze single-taste drugs is difficult, but to study and clarify the components and interactions in the compound Chinese prescriptions is more difficult. Doctors in China were not clear of the chemical components and structure of the root of wind-weed and gypsum; their experience told them that the two drugs were used as main ones when they applied them to the *Yangming* syndrome with flaring gastric heat accompanied by heat, thirst, profuse sweating and gigantic pulse to fight against pathogens and regain order. According to some Chinese medical theory, *Radix Anemarrhenae* and *Gypsum Fibrosum* are cold drugs for the treatment of the heat syndrome of excess type, and medical analysis and reduction show that *Radix Anemarrhenae* has many kinds of steroid saponins, which, hydrolyzed, produce *salso genin sapogenin*, a kind of substance containing nicotinic acid. As such, we are now clear about the heat-eliminating and sedation mechanism of *Radix Anemarrhenae*. The main component of *Gypsum Fibrosum* is hydrous calcium sulfate, which suppresses the heat-producing center and eliminates heat; at the same time, calcium acts as a sedative and anti-inflammatory element by inhibiting the neuromuscles and reducing the vascular permeability. Such scientific information is no doubt valuable for the use and study of Chinese drugs. However, analysis and reduction cannot reveal the full value of Chinese medicinal drugs. For instance, *Radix Anemarrhenae* and *Gypsum Fibrosum* are the principal drugs along with liquorice root and nonglutinous rice in the decoction *baihutang* which cures *Yangming* gastric heat syndrome. If ginseng is added, it will be able to replenish *qi* and produce clear body fluid; if bamboo leaf, it will be a recuperating recipe for the later stage of febrile disease patients in the later stages. Adding *Ramulus Cinnamomi* will harmonize and nurture the body to cure malaria, while *Rhizoma*

Atractylodis will cure rheumatic arthritis with fever and acute pain. *Baihutang* is often used to treat summer heat, acute gastroenteritis, vomiting and diarrhea. Such patients, suffering also from attack by external pathogenic factors, may be cured by adding *Herba Elsholtziae seu Moslae* and *Folium Perillae* to the principal decoction. Spasm of the gastrocnemius muscles with extreme heat (but appearing as if it were cold) should be treated by supplementing the decoction with *Herba Asari* and *Radix Clematidis*. For obstruction by phlegm, add *Cortex Magnoliae Officinalis* and *Rhizoma Pinelliae*, but for deficiency of blood and internal heat, add *Radix Rehmanniae* and *Cortex Lycii Radicis*. The addition of *Rhizoma Atractylodis Macrocephalae* and *Semen Coicis* will cure deficiency of *qi* in the spleno-gastric cavity. *Fructus Zizyphi Jujubae* and *Fructus Lycii* will cure patients debilitated by disease with short breath and letharg. Some people use *Radix Anemarrhenae* and *Gypsum Fibrosum* as the principal drugs and add *Semen Armeniacae Amarum*, *Cortex Magnolicae Officinalis*, *Radix Scutellariae* and *Radix Paeoniae Alba* to cure dampness, heat and white dysentery. Only by observing the traditional Chinese principles, methods, prescriptions and medicament can you get clear about the rich scientific contents and pharmacological actions between the drugs and body.

Obviously, anatomy, analysis and reduction are not main methods of getting Chinese medicine modernized and combined with Western medicine, though they may help discover the contents of Chinese drugs. It is only under the guidance of the theories and methods of the holistic system of traditional Chinese medicine that they become valuable. Some people fail to pay attention to this basic difference, and their interest and belief in Western science make them sure that the best choice is to combine clear, concise and reliable diagnostic techniques and knowledge of Western physiology and pathology with traditional Chinese medicine.

Some doctors give the powder *xiaoyaosan* to the

hepatitis patient, a Chinese drug used to treat hepatic and splenic diseases as soon as their diagnosis is confirmed. Drugs like *Rhizoma Coptidis*, *Radix Scutellariae* and *Fructus Forsythiae* are prescribed for a patient with inflammation, but *Radix Ginseng*, *Radix Astragalius* and other drugs are given to a patient feeling weak to invigorate the nervous and pituitary systems and improve the metabolism. These treatments, however, are seldom successful; Chinese medicine and drugs cannot be used according to Western medical theories. Chinese medical theories and methods cannot be overlooked or discarded, nor can the Chinese theoretical system. This kind of Chinese-Western combination will lead to the blind alley of "the Western use of Chinese drugs." As you know, such a method came in failure when it was introduced into Japan after the Meiji reform. There are other worse cases. Attention should be given to contraindications when using *baihutang* compounded with *Radix Anemarrhenae* and *Gypsum Fibrosum*, as warned by Wu Tang and another famous doctor Zhang Xichun (1860-1933). This decoction should not be given to a patient with his pulse floating, tense, short and deep, or one with his pulse floating but his external disease not relieved, or one who is thirsty and does not sweat. As there are no such prohibitive stipulations in Western medical patterns, Chinese drugs, if used in the style of Western medicine but not in conformity with Chinese medical theories and methods, will have little effect upon a disease. In worse cases, the nature of syndromes is not clear and contraindications are neglected. That is why a doctor cannot find out the reason of a disease— cold or heat, deficiency or excess, inside or outside, and yin or yang, treating a cold syndrome with cooling drugs and a heat syndrome with warming drugs, or curing an external disease internally and internal disease externally or making the deficiency sysndrome more deficient and excess syndrome more excessive. In so doing, the balance of yin and yang are further upset, the body's order further disturbed and the disease became more serious.

The tragedy is actually caused by "abolishing Chinese medicine while preserving Chinese drugs." The modernization of Chinese medicine and its combination with Western medicine are therefore dealt a setback. The more people are anxious to realize modernization and combination, the more they advocate Western diagnosis and Chinese treatment. With that the theories and methods of the Chinese medical science will be discarded, their therapeutic effects be neglected, and their side-effects be great. The lack of study of Chinese medicine in recent years and that of trained Chinese doctors have given rise to misapprehensions. Some people have gone in the opposite direction, maintaining that the lack was the result of combination and modernization. Others hold that Chinese medicine is the business of its professionals only and that there is no need for interference from other departments of science. This is insular thinking: no science is an exclusive system, but instead constantly absorbs new knowledge from other sciences and thereby develops. Traditional Chinese medicine itself has been continually replenished first by pre-Qin Dynasty scholars, and later by gathering many useful theories, techniques and drugs from foreign countries. So the most important is not whether we combine Chinese medicine with Western one or modernize Chinese medicine. What we are now in need of are an accurate understanding of combination and modernization and a correct approach to our aim.

The theoretical system and methodology of traditional Chinese medicine have every reason to occupy a high place in Chinese medical science. In this regard, Professor Manfred Porkert says in his book *The Difficult Task of Blending Chinese and Western Science: The Case of Modern Interpretations of Traditional Chinese Medicine*:

> Traditional Chinese medicine belongs to a category quite different from Western medical science. It is a science which is very rich in content, and is very

orderly and effective. Up to now, only a very small part of its therapeutic potential has been unearthed. At the moment, we have the three following imperative tasks to undertake:

A. Conveying to a top-notch crew of Chinese research scholars a clear grasp of the epistemology pertinent to the methodological amplification and adaptation of traditional Chinese medicine with respect to modern science. At first this task will probably have to be undertaken through cooperation between Chinese and Western scholars, since, to all evidence, in today's China not even the germ of such investigations seems to be in evidence.

B. Widely laying open the storehouse of the medical tradition. This task is directly dependent upon A but can and should essentially be undertaken by Chinese scholars. In spite of the critical inroads on classical philology before and during the cultural revolution, we are confident that China will rapidly recover sufficient qualified talent to develop this specific kind of qualification required to thoroughly explore the literary legacy of medical writers accumulated since Han times. Such investigation requires a double proficiency, viz. conversancy with classical and semi-classical texts as well as good grounding in Chinese and Western medical theory.

C. The systematic development of modern techniques. Traditional Chinese medicine, although it has brought forth some outstanding scientific talents, through the ages has been a practice-oriented discipline. Since the 19th century, and certainly for the past two decades, all consistent effort to elaborate new general or elementary techniques has practically come to a halt. From a deeper understanding of the rationale and the quality of the basic insights of traditional Chinese medicine, it will certainly be necessary and possible to develop, for instance, a new technique for developing and assaying new drugs, techniques for introducing or rejecting operative aids into function diagnostics; and certainly a general shakedown and checkup of the methodology and procedures of traditional Chinese medicine in view of the treatment of functional or degenerative ailments hitherto not covered in medical literature. This work again, I hope, will be done with the widest international cooperation since— I need not explain— such progress must not be restricted to one country only.

Porkert also believes that Chinese medical theory must be grasped in terms of scientific methodology of Chinese medicine before Chinese medicine can be used and modern technology can be systematically developed. Although it is now more necessary than ever before to do research into Chinese medicine by means of modern science and technology, its modernization must be based on its own theories and methods. New methods will surely come from modern science and technology to explain and supplement Chinese theories and methods. Strategically, we must also develop these theories and methods through dialectical materialism and modern scientific methods like cybernetics, informatics and systematics. We should not discard the essence of Chinese medical theories and methods or pay too much attention to the Western methods of dissection, analysis and reduction to make Chinese medicine modernized.

The Training of Chinese Medical Personnel

"The past is prologue," says the Chinese proverb. A review of the history of medical education in China will prove useful here.

In ancient China, medical education was offered in government institutes such as the Imperial Academy of

Medicine, but the number of professionals trained there was too small to meet the needs of the masses. For this reason, a task fell on the society to train a large number of professionals by way of apprenticeship or the transmission of the medical art from father to son, as in the ancient handicraft industries. Although this transmission had many defects, it did enjoy one strong point: the apprentices, from the first day of training, were under the step-by-step guidance of the masters. Apprentices learned how to make diagnosis, give treatment and prepare prescriptions with the presence of the patient so that they could learn about the treating effects themselves. This way of training doctors has existed in China for ages and helped bring up a large number of medical workers, given its vast territory and large population. Doctors specialized in traditional medicine are familiar with the locality, the seasons and the climate, and know what disease is prevalent in some specific regions as well as the cause of diseases and the living conditions of patients. Besides, they are able to observe the prognostic development, the changes and the therapeutic effects of the medicines. It is from their work that many doctors have broadened the frontiers of their knowledge about Chinese medicine. All this makes it possible to have traditional Chinese medicine developed over the years.

These ancient methods are better suited to Chinese medicine that is full of natural philosophical ideas. It enjoys a broad and integral theoretical system, though abstract, conceptually generalized and comparatively vague and ambiguous in its theories, which tend to relate the "hows" but not the "whys". Only when people have had enough experience can they find out the value and meaning of the principles, methods, prescriptions and drugs used in Chinese medicine and make use of them skilfully. Feeling the pulse, for one, is a method of diagnosis in Chinese medicine. Those who have just started to learn Chinese medicine would feel perceptible in mind but uncertain at the fingers even though they keep in mind the main passages of classical books on pulsation. Qian Xuesen said on one occasion, "A student of Chinese medicine cannot work as a doctor on his own when he has just mastered the theory; he has to be coached by his master when he gives treatment. It is usually three or four years before he begins to work by himself. He can become a qualified doctor in his right when he has had enough experience in clinical diagnosis." Chinese medicine is not so standardized as those of Western medicine in diagnosis and treatment. It is a large and all-inclusive system of theories and methods. Without careful study and repeated practice, there will hardly be a comprehensive understanding of its essence.

Having perused ancient and modern history by means of dialectic and historical materialism, Chinese historian Fan Wenlan (1893-1969) had this to say about his experience, "There are rational components in old things, and old things cannot be one hundred percent perfect when they are brought into being. Old things will not perish unless they are absolutely obsolete, while it will be difficult for new things to replace the old unless they are completely matured and incorporate all the strong points of the old. This is especially true of cultural phenomena." We should draw upon what is useful in the old and constantly improve the new Chinese medical education.

A large number of students have graduated from medical colleges and schools in China since 1949. However, we lack experience managing advanced programs and schools, and have done very little to absorb past experience in medical education and in studying the laws and characteristic features of traditional Chinese medicine itself. Therefore, although college education developed rapidly in many different districts, the methods adopted were almost the same as those in Western medical education. It was therefore difficult to build colleges and schools of traditional medicine in a practical and realistic way.

Students are now required to take many courses in theory, so they have little time to take part in practice, still less treat patients under the tutelage of their teachers. This state of affairs can also be found in lectures on such basic texts as *Shang Han Lun* and *Jin Kui Yao Lue Fang Lun*. These works, dealing with theories and methods of treatment on the basis of *bianzheng*, should be included in clinical courses and combined with practice; as a matter of fact they are only explained in the classroom. No wonder graduates from those schools are often bewildered and at a loss what to do when they are told to treat patients on their own. They have to rely on the description of the tastes of drugs and the precis of treatments in some medical works, randomly picking out the standard drugs or ways of treatment. As a result, their treatment is not effective.

Some graduate students complain that Chinese medicine is not standardized and difficult to master. They therefore attempt to use the meager knowledge of Western medicine they learned at college. Research shows that many graduates change their profession every year, which makes trained doctors in Chinese medicine fewer and fewer. That is why the most important now is to have educational reform in Chinese medicine. Here are some of my points of view.

First, adopt the walking-on-two-leg policy[25]. This requires us to improve the management of regular colleges and schools of traditional Chinese medicine and encourage a practicable and effective meththod of learning traditional medicine by means of apprenticeship. But this does not only mean the restoration of the old pattern; instead, something new is added and the management strengthened to ensure the quality of future doctors. For this aim, regulations are formulated and examinations conducted on professional expertise and clinical techniques. Those who stand the tests are awarded a degree equal to those who graduate from university. In addition, medical college graduates are allowed to set up their own clinics by themselves or in partnership with others. All these measures may help bring up a large number of medical workers with genuine talent and solid knowledge on the one hand and encourage more young people to take a course in traditional medicine and set up a reserve of Chinese doctors for the future on the other.

Secondly, encourage students to take part in medical activities. To this aim, conditions are created for students in the first year of college to help their teachers or doctors with work so that they can get a clear picture of diseases themselves by combining theory with practice. Only when a solid foundation is laid can the development of Chinese medicine be guaranteed. As you know, laboratory is a principal basis in Western medicine for teaching and learning and research. Chinese medicine, however, uses as its main method the input of information into human body and the analysis of the output on the basis of physiology, pathology and pharcaceutical properties. Therefore, clinical observation, treatment and the on-going improvement of therapeutic methods are of special significance in its development. We can say that those who have contributed much to the advancement of Chinese medicine are all good doctors. They combine modern theories and techniques with those of traditional medicine in their work, and to get Chinese medicine modernized like this is in conformity with the Chinese system as advocated by some people.

Hospitals need to be established under medical colleges and schools so as to offer students with an opportunity for clinical observation and practice. Besides, help from local hospitals and private clinics is also necessary, and in return teachers and doctors are sent from colleges to give advice in these institutions. In so doing, they help develop traditional Chinese medicine. This will not only ease the lack of places for practice but raise the theoretical and technical level of local hospitals and private clinics.

Thirdly, make the structure of medical workers' knowledge better meet the needs of the situation and carry on educational reform. About the structure of knowledge, Engels wrote in *Dialektik und Natur*:

Motion, in the most general sense, conceived as the mode of existence, the inherent attribute, of matter, comprehends all changes and processes occurring in the universe, from mere change of place right to thinking. The investigation of the nature of motion had as a matter of course to start from the lowest, simplest forms of this motion and to learn to grasp these before it could achieve anything in the way of explanation of the higher and more complicated forms. Hence, in the historical evolution of the natural sciences we see how first of all the theory of simplest change of place, the mechanics of heavenly bodies and terrestrial masses, was developed; it was followed by the theory of molecular motion, physics, and immediately afterwards, almost alongside of it and in some places in advance of it, the science of the motion of atoms, chemistry. Only after these different branches of the knowledge of the forms of motion governing non-living nature had attained a high degree of development could the explanation of the process of motion represented by the life process be successfully tackled. This advanced in proportion with the progress of mechanics, physics and chemistry.

The study of each type of higher motion uses, as its basis, the series of lower types. To understand and study biology, which reflects the motion of life, one needs to understand the motion of mechanics, physics and chemistry. Therefore, to be a biologist, in addition to biology itself, one should also have a background in mathematics, mechanics, physics and chemistry. The mastery of medical science, which studies the physiology and pathology of the human body and the prevention and treatment of diseases, therefore also demands some rudimentary knowledge of the natural sciences. In the past, Western medicine studied the human body mainly from the angle of biology, neglecting social and psychological factors. This was understandable at a time when science was in its early stages, and biological medicine could reflect the substance of the human in society and displaying its mental activities. Efforts are now being made to develop the pattern of biological medicine into a social-psychological-biological pattern, expanding medical knowledge and placing it in a much wider, multi-disciplinary field. It is expected that this will result in further methodological reform.

Along with these general requirements, there are also special requirements of Chinese medicine that spring from specific foundation of Chinese civilization and are closely related to Chinese philosophy as well as such natural sciences as ancient astronomy, meteorology, and calendar calculation. For instance, Confucianism, Budhhism and Taoism have to a certain degree permeated Chinese medicine. The *liujing*, *liuqi* and *ziwuliuzhu* theories owe much to astronomy, geography, meteorology, and study of the seasons and time. These provide basis for such comprehensive theoretical systems as those which trace the relationship between man and nature, *zang* and *xiang*, body and spirit, and men and society. Consequently, advanced Chinese medical workers must also understand Chinese culture and science. Chinese philosophical thought, ancient natural science and culture are significant for the understanding of the principles, methods, prescriptions and medicament of traditional medicine, and the explanation of its academic system. To attain this objective, it is necessary for colleges and research institutes to develop a system for six or seven years of training; a special system may also be instituted, offering bachelor's and master's degrees and, for postgraduates the doctoral degree.

Education in ordinary medical colleges may keep the present five-year system, but curricular reform should be introduced. Redundant courses should be simplified and eliminated to allow time for courses on the history of Chinese culture, medical methodology, introduction to natural sciences, medical psychology, and the theory and practice of *qigong*, for instance.

There is a need of bringing up qualified pharmacologists in China. This may be done through the combination of traditional Chinese and modern methods. In addition, more colleges of Chinese pharmacology should be set up across the country and departments of pharmacology opened in Chinese medical colleges, so that the long-proven superiority of biological drugs will be displayed.

China has a population of one billion, of which 800 million are peasants. It is therefore necessary to train a large group of university and college students over two or three years to meet the needs of countryside and border areas. The education of these students should aim chiefly to give them the ability to treat and prevent diseases and protect health in accordance with the basic Chinese theory and methodology. Study of additional subjects is also advised if the situation allows.

A good basis has been laid for compiling teaching materials for hospitals and colleges since 1949. Efforts should be doubled to promote higher quality with less duplication of materials that embody Chinese medicine and pharmacology and assimilate related accomplishments of modern science.

An important tendency of world medical science aims at mobilizing the body's own ability to protect health and treat diseases, as well as non-traumatic treatments and cures. This is a principle that has been observed in Chinese medicine for ages. And *qigong* has been found valuable for the improvement of health and treatment of diseases and the development of body's potential. Moreover, with the development of economy and the raising of living standards, the average life span of the Chinese people has been extended. This makes gerontology all the more important. *Qigong* plays an important part in the development of the medical science, so we have every reason to get *qigong* theories and exercises systematized, prepare teaching materials and train instructors for such a course.

As the first step, symposiums and lectures are held in traditional hospitals and medical institutes in order to make *qigong* more popular than ever before. A number of suggestions have been offered, and one of them is to have several hours of *qigong* practice in the PE course in medical colleges so that students can master its skills at college.

Methodology cannot be overemphasized in the development of Chinese medicine. In addition to a generalization of traditional theories and methods, methodology should also use include dialectic materialism as its guid and draw on systematics, cybernetics and informatics along with mathematical methods.

At present the main objective of hospitals and medical institutes is to train students for work in general medicine, while surgery, orthopedics, bone injury, anorectology, gynecology, ophthalmology, nasopharyngology, otology, acupuncture-moxibustion, massage, *qigong* exercises, nutrition and other specialized departments receive little attention. This does not benefit the traditional specialities offered in medical departments or meet the needs of common people. It is therefore suggested that medical establishments be grouped according to geographical location where departments or advanced classes are opened to train specialized doctors.

The Promotion of Research and Practice

The development of science depends on research and practice; they must be doubled if Chinese medicine is to be modernized. Two jobs should be done in research: succession and renovation.

Chinese medicine started its existence 2,000-3,000 years ago, and what is included in it has become rich. However, ideas were quite conservative in the feudal and semi-feudal and semi-colonial societies. Special skills and knowledge were usually seen as family heirlooms and could not be made known to the public or even exchanged in the same trade. Moreover, the ancient mecdical classics were difficult to decipher; to get a good grasp of them, you have to deliberate and practice again and again. That is why Chinese medicine is not so popular and even lost in part. Following the semi-colonization of China, the traditional medical theories and techniques were repudiated by some portions of the populace, which also harmed the treasury of Chinese medicine. As a result, in redeveloping Chinese medicine, much work still remains to explore and revive this treasury. The classics must be systematized and annotated, and lost or dispersed literature must be located and collected. The experience of well-known doctors has to be compiled, elucidated and commented upon, and the academic thought of doctors from various schools and dynasties needs to be studied. Moreover, standardization of the terminology of diseases, syndromes and diagnoses is also an indispensable part of research The successful accomplishment of these tasks will enable the rich history and practical experience of traditional Chinese medicine to serve the development of modern medical science.

In addition to summarizing the experience acquired during medical treatment, the study of the multiple disciplines of Chinese medicine is the key to development and modernization. Chinese medicinehas developed historically by absorbing related multi-disciplinary thought and technology. Today, we are more in need of modernmulti-displinary achievements. In recent years, despite enthusiastic and painstaking multi-disciplinary research, the magnitude of the volume of work and methodological problems have impeded major breakthroughs; the advance has also been slowed by misconceptions.

Therefore, we should once again raise the problem of methodology. As mentioned above, Chinese and Western medicine deals with different academic systems developed under different social and historical conditions. They study physiology and pathology and the prevention and treatment of diseases from different angles, and in addition employ different theories and methods. In the past, due to a lack of sufficient understanding of this fundamental difference, Western theories and methods have been unconsciously employed to conduct scientific research in Chinese medicine. For instance, anatomical measures have been used to study the theories of *jingluo* and *zang* and *fu*; cytopathology to study *bianzhenglunzhi*; and methods of simple analysis and chemical examination to study Chinese pharmacology. Such methods are helpful in solving local problems or particulars; but unless Chinese medicine is studied as a holistic system, this merely amounts to the research of Western medicine using Chinese medicine and pharmacology as an objective. Moreover, if such methods are regarded as absolute and used improperly, that would mean that you stretch on the procrustean bed. That may explain in part why some in Chinese and Western medical circles show have little understanding of each other and even harbor mutual distrust.

Do not forget the holistic nature of Chinese medicine when you adapt Western methods for Chinese use. In Chinese physiology, pathology, and prevention and treatment, the action of one factor or law in a holistic system upon the other and any change in their relationships afford a basis for Chinese physiology, pathology and methods of prevention and treatment.

To raise the level of health maintenance and clinical treatment is of course important because of its role in promoting traditional medicine and meeting the growing demand of the masses for improved prevention and treatment. But that cannot take the place of basic researches, especialy those conducted in the laboratory. Animal models are useful in research but much different from the human body. If working directly on human physiology and disease prevention and treatment with the help of Chinese medical theories and methods, a doctor will discover something more interesting and practical. For instance, the *jingluo* theory and the effects of acupuncture and moxibustion upon diseases became clear when a method like opening the black box was used on the body.

This makes it necessary to consider the problem of whether a single therapeutic case should be regarded as an accomplishment of scientific research. In recent years, it has even been stipulated in some regions that case reports with fewer than 50 or 100 instances cannot be regarded as scientific, since a single case is liable to show unusual results. This is not completely in conformity with the *bianzhenglunzhi* principle, whose basis is the interaction between the human body and pathogenic factors of the internal and external environments. Due to such interrelated factors as pathogens, the patient's constitution, internal and external environments, and identical diseases often show different syndromes, while different diseases may show identical syndromes. Accordingly, Chinese treatment cannot be stereotyped into fixed formulas or standardized. In composing prescriptions, administering drugs and readjusting their components, multiple factors must be considered, such as the principal syndrome and the subsidiary syndromes and their development of trends, the patient's constitution, the season and the climate, the locality and environment. Obviously, Chinese medical treatment cannot be standardized like that of Western medicine, which administers unified prescriptions after having identified the cause, the site and the pathology of the disease. In the case of Chinese medicine, there are great differences in the scope and depth of the art and technique of identifying and treating diseases; every single case records the ever-changing conditions of the diseases and the fluctuations of the internal and external environments. This reflects clinical thinking and methodology of physicians, their knowledge and principles of treatiment, their practical experience, their academic thought, comprehension and mastery of the regularities of treatment. Therefore, their case reports contain many guiding and enligtening significant ideas. Ye Tianshi, for one, left not only a voluminous theoretical work, but also a collection of medical case records, representing his lifetime experience in medical treatment. Many of his case histories show his incisive understanding and judicious judgment of febrile diseases; we certainly cannot overlook such case records, and should indeed rely more on their contents.

In evaluating clinical research, the characteristic features of Chinese medicine should also be considered. The cytopathological theory of Rudolf Virchow, formulated by employing Western methods of anatomy, analysis and reduction, still exercises a profound influence on the evaluative criterion of clinical cures. Western medicine as such relies mostly on the elimination of pathological changes in local tissues and cells. For instance, the shrinkage or disappearance of cancer cells in the lungs is taken as the principal indicator of a turn for the better or a cure of pulmonary cancer. Chinese medical treatment, on the other hand, starts from the holistic system of human body to readjust its relative equilibrium of yin and yang and the order of *zang* and *fu* organs, and to restore its ability to resist diseases and cure itself. In the case of a lung cancer patient, a condition may ensue after Chinese medical treatment when the cancer cells are inhibited and restrained by the organism, thus basically eliminating the syndrome. Such therapeutic effect should of course be accorded scientific evaluation. Moreover, if we go forward and study the mechanism in which such disease is controlled and health restored, it is entirely possible that we might be able to discover a new field of medical science and uncover its scientific mystery. Isn't this precisely what the development of modern immunology has done, clarifying some mechanisms of Chinese medicine and presenting new and valuable thoughts for treatment?

Some hospitals devote time not only to health maintenance and medical treatment but also to medical training and research. Therefore, a network of such hospitals should be formed to give advice and coordinate work, with towns and cities playing a key role but the countryside given priority for development. This makes it possible for the masses to enjoy fine medical treatment and for hospitals and colleges of Chinese medicine to have training bases.

The development of Chinese medicine is a "big system" dealing with many fields, and our aim is to have a developmental principle in this chapter, or for that matter, in the whole book. That is what I have pursued all my life, and I am willing to do everything I can to make it true, and the present book is just an attempt. But due to my scanty knowledge and experience, there are quite a few defects and shortcomings in my work. Anyway, I have cast out brick in hope of attracting jade.

NOTES

1 *Cun* and *chi* are two of the three places on the wrist over the radial artery to feel the pulse, the third being *guan* (bar) just over the eminent head of the radius at the wrist, where the tip of the physician's middle finger is placed. *Cun* is next to it on the distal side, where the tip of the physician's index finger rests. *Chi* is on the proximal side where the tip of the physician's ring finger is placed. *Cun, guan* and *chi* on the left represent the pulse condition of the heart, liver and kidney respectively while those on the right represent the pulse condition of the lung, spleen and *mingmen* (vital gate).

2 The *renying* pulse at the area lateral to the laryngeal prominence in the neck, where the common carotid pulsatations can be felt.

3 The *fuyang* pulse, the dorsal pedal pulsations palpable at the *chongyang* point, on the dorsum of the foot four or five centimeters distal to the ankle crease, between two tendons.

4 The body is divided into three regions— the head, the upper limbs and the lower limbs. Each region has three sets of arteries – the upper, the middle and the lower— with a total of nine nodes of pulsations for the entire body.

5 See note 4.

6 In Chinese it is *fa*, meaning law. Here it indicates the principle of treatment to various diseases, or the methodology.

7 *Zangxiang* is a theory on physiological activities and pathological changes of internal and external organs, etc., and their interrelations.

8 For instance, the invention of the microscope, by the Dutch scientist Antonie van Leeuwenhoek (1632-1723), played a major role in promoting the development of the theory of microstructure in the tissues of the human body and in microbiology.

9 When a word standing for an internal organ, say liver, it just means a system but not a liver as said in anatomy.

10 *Zang* includes the heart, liver, spleen, lung and kidney, while *fu* mesns gallbladder, stomach, large intestine, small intestine, urinary bladder and triple energizer, and they will be referred to as *zang* and *fu* in the rest of the book unless there is a special explanation.

11 Traditional Chinese medicine combines the theory of *wuyun* with the changes of the six kinds of climate (wind, cold, damp-heat, dampness, dryness and fire) to explain the relationship between changes in the weather and the incidence of disease in the body.

12 *Ziwuliuzhu* is a theory of acupuncture in ancient China.

13 *Bagua*, consisting of eight combinations of three solid or broken lines used in divination, symbolizes the changing balance of forces.

14 *Wuxing* refers to the five elements of metal, wood, water, fire and

earth. It was believed to be part and parcel of the physical universe first in ancient China and then used in traditional Chinese medicine to explain various physiological and pathological phenomena.

15 See *Huang Di Nei Jing*

16 *Liujing* refers to the six of the 12 main channels in traditional Chinese medicine, namely *Taiyin, Shaoyin, Jueyin, Yangming, Taiyang* and *Shaoyang*.

17 *Wuqi* means *qi* (vital energy) coming from the five-*zang* organs.

18 *Wuwei* refers to the five kinds of flavor, namely pungent, sweet, sour, bitter and salty.

19 *Wuse* refers to the five colors, namely blue, yellow, red, white and black.

20 *Wusheng* refers to the five kinds of sound, shouting, laughing, singing, wailing and groaning.

21 These terms denote the four portions or strata of the body from the superficial to the deep to show the location and seriousness or stages of a febrile disease as a guide to diagnosis.

22 *Zi, chou, yin, mao, chen, si, wu, wei, shen, you, xu* and *hai* are the twelve earth branches in China and can be used to designate the hours of a day, with *zi* standing for 23:00-1:00, *chou* for 1:00-3:00, *yin* for 3:00-5:00, *mao* for 5:00-7:00, *chen* for 7:00-9:00, *si* for 9:00-11:00, *wu* for 11:00-13:00, *wei* for 13:00-15:00, *shen* for 15:00-17:00, *you* for 17:00-19:00, *xu* for 19:00-21:00 and *hai* for 21:00-23:00.

23 The six *zang* organs refer to the heart, liver, spleen, lung, kidney and pericardium.

24 The decoction *baihutang* consists of *Gypsum Gibrosum, Rhizoma Anemarrhenae, Radix Glycyrrhizae* and *Semon Oryzae Nonglutinosae*.

25 A common saying in China, which at first referred to a series of government policies for balancing the relations between industry and agriculture, and heavy and light industry, but now means that two or more methods should be employed when you try to do something important.

INDEX

Aishibi, 47
Albert Szent-Gyorgyi, 97, 164
Alexandria Period, 153
Andreas Vesalius, 10
August Kekule von Stradonitz, 45

Bagua, 22, 23
Ben Cao Bei Yao, 37
Ben Cao Gang Mu, 37, 58
Bian Que, 81
Bianzheng, 106, 108, 109, 110, 111, 112, 114, 124
Bianzhenglunzhi, 9, 14, 20, 21, 39, 105, 108, 122, 152, 162, 182, 183
Black box, 17, 18, 19, 20, 32, 35, 75, 76, 80, 84, 101, 123, 124, 129, 165, 166, 183
Bladder Channel of Foot-*Taiyang*, 54, 55
Budhhism, 178

Chedd, 12, 13
Chen Jiewen, 63
Chinese Medicine— A Miracle in the History of Sciences, 47
Christian Era, 153
Chunfen, 52
Confucianism, 42, 178

Dantian, 41
Dao, 22, 24, 39
Deficiency, 20, 26, 33, 34, 36, 61, 62, 63, 64, 65, 66, 68, 88, 90, 97, 109, 115, 117, 130, 135, 137, 138, 140, 142, 144, 145, 146, 147, 149, 150, 151, 166, 168, 169
Design of the Cerebrum, 47
Dialektik und Natur, 18, 155, 176

Dongzhi, 52, 53
Du channel, 54, 81

Eastern Han Dynasty, 72, 105
Electrobiology and Cancer, 97, 164
Ernst Mach, 5
Excess, 20, 26, 33, 34, 63, 69, 92, 109, 130, 135, 142, 143, 144, 146, 147, 166, 167, 169
Expand the Basic Research in the Science of the Human Body, 83

Fan Wenlan, 174
Francis Bacon, 10
Fredrich Engels, 8, 9, 12, 18, 52, 155, 176
Fu, 14, 30, 31, 34, 38, 54, 71, 84, 85, 86, 87, 90, 91, 93, 94, 96, 98, 99, 100, 101, 104, 105, 110, 131, 138, 139, 141, 182, 184

Gallbladder Channel of Foot-*Shaoyang*, 55
Goldberg, 23
Gottfried Wilhelm Leibniz, 22, 23

Han Dynasty, 6, 24, 71, 72, 95, 103
Han Shu, 71
Heart Channel of Hand-*Shaoyin*, 55
Hippocratic School, 153
Hou Han Shu, 72
Hua Guofan, 47
Hua Tuo, 72
Hua Yang Zang Fu Tu Xiang Yue Zuan, 165
Huai Nan Zi, 103
Huang Di Nei Jing, 24, 25, 26, 27, 30, 31, 37, 39, 42, 44, 45, 46,

53, 56, 61, 68, 71, 74, 75, 81, 84, 91, 92, 93, 95, 96, 97, 102, 104, 105, 113, 117, 119, 137, 138, 139, 142, 154, 165

Jin Dynasty, 36
Jin Guantao, 47
Jin Kui Yao Lue, 132
Jin Kui Yao Lue Fang Lun, 32, 51, 146, 175
Jing, 14, 30, 40, 71, 80, 85, 91, 92, 93, 94, 96, 97, 99, 141, 142
Jingluo, 14, 19, 20, 35, 40, 54, 55, 71, 74, 79, 80, 81, 82, 89, 96, 98, 99, 100, 126, 139, 158, 159, 182, 183
John Locke, 10

Kidney Channel of Foot-*Shaoyin*, 55

Large Intestine Channel of Hand-*Yangming*, 55
Li Dongyuan, 36, 38
Li Gao, 143
Li Shizhen, 58, 80, 82
Liu An, 103
Liujing, 27, 28, 53, 108, 110, 111, 130, 133, 178
Liuqi, 14, 25, 28, 53, 124, 125, 127, 178
Liver Channel of Foot-*Jueyin*, 55
Louis Pasteur, 117, 123
Ludwig von Bertalanffy, 15, 163
Lun Heng, 95
Lung Channel of Hand-*Taiyin*, 55, 141

Manfred Porkert, 160, 170, 172
Mao Zedong, 160
Marxism, 79
Mawangdui, 81
Middle Ages, 153
Ming Dynasty, 80

Nan Jing, 45, 50, 105
New Medicine and Pharmacy Journal, 61
New Science, 12

Norbert Wiener, 16
N. D. Cook, 65

Pathogenic factors, 20, 32, 34, 49, 69, 70, 96, 106, 107, 108, 110, 114, 117, 118, 119, 122, 123, 124, 127, 128, 142, 143, 144, 145, 146, 149, 150, 168, 183
People's Daily, 59
Pericardium Channel of Hand-*Jueyin*, 55
Period of Warring States, 81, 105

Qi, 14, 19, 20, 25, 26, 28, 30, 31, 34, 35, 39, 40, 41, 55, 56, 70, 71, 73, 74, 80, 81, 82, 83, 84, 87, 89, 92, 93, 94, 95, 96, 97, 98, 99, 101, 108, 109, 110, 111, 112, 113, 115, 117, 118, 119, 120, 121, 122, 125, 126, 128, 130, 132, 135, 138, 139, 140, 141, 142, 158, 167, 168
Qi Huan Hou, 81
Qi Jing Ba Mai Kao, 80
Qian Jin Yao Fang, 116, 141
Qian Xuesen, 16, 83, 161, 163
Qin Dynasty, 24, 52, 104, 170
Qing Dynasty, 37, 79, 149, 165
Qiufen, 52

Ren channel, 54, 81
Renaissance, 154, 156
Resistance, 32, 34, 78, 112, 117, 118, 120, 122, 124, 128, 142, 143, 144, 149
Robert Koch, 123
Roman Empire, 153
Rudolf Virchow, 10, 11, 184
R. Rosen, 163

Shang Dynasty, 104
Shang Fang, 71
Shang Han Lun, 27, 32, 56, 85, 105, 110, 111, 133, 175
Shang Han Za Bing Lun, 105
Shen Nong, 103
Shen Nong Ben Cao, 103
Shi Ji, 81
Siqi, 37, 38, 97, 166

189

Small Intestine Channel of Hand-Taiyang, 55
Song Shu, 72
Southern Dynasties, 72
Spleen Channel of Foot-*Taiyin*, 55
Spring and Autumn Period, 105
Stomach Channel of Foot-*Yangming*, 55, 56, 90
Sun Simiao, 116, 141

Tang Ci, 72
Tang Dynasty, 74
Tang Zonghai, 165
Taoism, 178
Technology of Organization Management— Systems Engineering, 16
The Difficult Task of Blending Chinese and Western Science: The Case of Modern Interpretation of Traditional Chinese Medicine, 170
The Journal of Traditional Chinese Medicine, 78
The Seven Books on the Structure of the Human Body, 10
Trio-*Jiao* Channel of Hand-*Shaoyang*, 55
Triple energizer, 108, 111, 112, 113
Tuna, 40, 41

Wang Ang, 37
Wang Bing, 74
Wang Chong, 95
Wang Shouyuan, 16
Wen Bing Tiao Bian, 113
Wen Hui Bao, 16
White box, 18
Wu Tang, 113
Wuqi, 28
Wuse, 28, 44, 50, 51, 75, 76
Wusheng, 28, 44, 50, 51, 75, 76
Wuwei, 28, 37, 38, 44, 50, 51, 97, 166
Wuxing, 24, 25, 27, 31, 32, 34, 35, 36, 42, 43, 44, 45, 46, 47, 48, 49, 50, 51, 52, 73, 91, 100, 104, 127, 139, 140, 158
Wuyun, 14, 28

Xia Zongqin, 66
Xiazhi, 52
Xiu Ruijuan, 98
Xu Guozhi, 16
Xu Lingtai, 149

Yang, 9, 14, 19, 20, 21, 22, 23, 24, 25, 26, 27, 28, 29, 30, 31, 32, 33, 34, 35, 36, 37, 38, 39, 40, 41, 46, 49, 50, 52, 53, 54, 56, 57, 59, 61, 62, 63, 64, 65, 66, 67, 68, 69, 70, 73, 75, 76, 84, 86, 87, 88, 90, 91, 94, 96, 97, 99, 100, 104, 105, 106, 109, 110, 111, 115, 116, 117, 118, 120, 121, 122, 124, 125, 126, 127, 128, 130, 133, 134, 135, 136, 137, 138, 139, 144, 145, 146, 147, 150, 152, 154, 166, 169, 184
Yang-*qi*, 37, 56, 69, 90, 96, 125, 126
Ye Tianshi, 112, 183
Yi Jing, 22, 23
Yin, 9, 14, 19, 20, 21, 22, 23, 24, 25, 26, 27, 28, 29, 30, 31, 32, 33, 34, 35, 36, 37, 38, 39, 40, 41, 46, 49, 50, 52, 53, 54, 56, 57, 59, 61, 62, 63, 65, 66, 67, 68, 73, 75, 76, 84, 86, 90, 91, 94, 96, 97, 99, 100, 104, 105, 106, 109, 110, 111, 113, 114, 115, 116, 117, 118, 120, 121, 122, 124, 125, 126, 127, 128, 130, 133, 134, 135, 136, 137, 138, 139, 144, 145, 146, 147, 149, 150, 151, 152, 154, 166, 169, 184
Yin Yang Shi Yi Mai Jiu Jing, 81
Yin-*qi*, 56, 96
Yin-yang theory, 9, 20, 22, 52, 84, 152

Zang, 14, 19, 21, 29, 30, 31, 32, 34, 38, 44, 47, 48, 49, 51, 54, 71, 72, 74, 75, 76, 84, 85, 86, 87, 89, 90, 91, 93, 94, 96, 98, 99, 100, 101, 104, 105, 110, 130, 131, 138, 139, 141, 178, 182, 184
Zangxiang, 9, 14, 19, 20, 48, 71, 73, 74, 75, 76, 78, 79, 82, 84, 86, 90, 98, 99, 100, 101, 104, 127, 130, 152, 154, 158, 165

Zang-fu organs, 14, 19, 20, 30, 35, 39, 40, 43, 44, 48, 49, 54, 65, 68, 71, 73, 74, 75, 79, 80, 85, 86, 87, 91, 92, 93, 94, 96, 98, 99, 108, 109, 110, 122, 125, 127, 130, 139, 140, 159
Zhang Jingyue, 46, 74, 143
Zhang Xiangtong, 100, 165
Zhang Xichun, 169
Zhang Zhongjing, 6, 31, 32, 56, 105, 133
Zhong Xi Yi Hui Tong Yi Jing Jing Yi, 165
Zhou Dynasty, 22, 42
Zhoutian, 81
Zhu Danxi, 144
Zhu Peiwen, 165
Ziwuliuzhu, 14, 28, 55, 56, 178
Zu Bi Shi Yi Mai Jiu Jing, 81
Zuo Shi Chun Qiu, 28

图书在版编目（CIP）数据

中医方法论：英文/黄建平著.
—北京：新世界出版社，1995.6
ISBN 7-80005-266-4

Ⅰ.中…
Ⅱ.黄…
Ⅲ.中国医药学-理论-研究-英文
Ⅳ.R2

中 医 方 法 论

黄建平 著

*

新世界出版社出版
（北京百万庄路 24 号）
北京大学印刷厂印刷
中国国际图书贸易总公司发行
（中国北京车公庄西路 35 号）
北京邮政信箱第 399 号　邮政编码 100044
1995 年(英文)第一版
ISBN 7-80005-266-4
02400
14-E-3015P